YOUR CHOICES MAKE THE DIFFERENCE IN DIABETES CONTROL. DID YOU KNOW?

***You can improve your health in just seven days . . .** A delicious meal plan—including snacks—helps melt away excess pounds and may reduce your insulin needs . . . starting today.

***You can trade your candy bars for a treadmill . . .** Regular, gentle exercise lowers blood sugar, raises energy levels *substantially*, and delivers other health benefits to boot.

***You don't have to feel deprived . . .** Delicious recipes abound for satisfying a sweet tooth without high doses of dangerous sugars.

***You can heal with herbs . . .** Nature's medicines contain an array of compounds that can prevent diabetes-related nerve damage, improve circulation, and more.

***You can combat syndrome X . . .** Trademark symptoms like insulin resistance and weight gain are no match for smart lifestyle choices.

***You don't have to hurt . . .** New testing methods take the "ouch" out of monitoring your blood sugar levels.

OUTSMART DIABETES

PREVENTION'S™

Outsmart Diabetes

Also by the Editors of *Prevention* Health Books

Outsmart High Cholesterol

Outsmart Arthritis

Outsmart High Blood Pressure

The Ice Cream Diet

The Peanut Butter Diet

Available from St. Martin's Paperbacks

PREVENTION'S™

Outsmart Diabetes

EXPERT-ENDORSED STRATEGIES FOR STAYING HEALTHY AND LIVING LONGER WITH DIABETES

The Editors of
Prevention Health Books

St. Martin's Paperbacks

PREVENTION'S OUTSMART DIABETES

ISBN: 0-312-98813-3

Printed in the United States of America

Rodale / St. Martin's Paperbacks edition / November 2003

St. Martin's Paperbacks are published by St. Martin's Press, 175 Fifth Avenue, New York, NY 10010.

10 9 8 7 6 5 4 3 2 1

NOTICE

This book is intended as a reference volume only, not as a medical manual. The information presented here is designed to help you make informed decisions about your health. It is not intended as a substitute for any treatment that may have been prescribed by your doctor. If you suspect that you have a medical problem, we urge you to seek competent medical care. If you have not participated in an exercise program regularly or recently, we encourage you to work with your physician to determine the activity level that is best for you.

Mention of specific companies, organizations, or authorities in this book does not imply endorsement by the publisher, nor does mention of specific companies, organizations, or authorities imply that they endorse the book.

Any Internet addresses and telephone numbers provided in this book were accurate at the time the book went to press.

CONTENTS

INTRODUCTION

If you or someone you love has been diagnosed with diabetes, you're far from alone. An estimated 17 million Americans are living with the disease. Yet only two-thirds of them know it. That's unfortunate, because in many cases, early intervention in the form of some simple lifestyle changes could make all the difference in effectively controlling blood sugar and avoiding serious complications.

Of course, the challenge of managing diabetes lies in knowing where to begin. The sheer volume of information can be overwhelming to sort through. That's exactly why we organized this book to be as simple and straightforward as possible. We set out to provide the very latest news from the frontline of diabetes research, as well as expert-recommended solutions for real-world diabetes management. Along the way, we share the true stories of people just like you who are fighting back against the disease, often against remarkable odds.

In Part I, you'll find answers to many of the questions that follow on the heels of a diabetes diagnosis: Just what is diabetes? How is it treated? Can it be prevented? What are its complications? If you don't yet have diabetes but you're concerned about getting the disease, you can take a simple quiz to assess your personal risk.

Part II introduces the latest tools and techniques for effective blood sugar control, as well as medical tests that are a vital component of any self-care plan. You'll get valuable pointers on how to avoid dangerous nighttime blood sugar dips and how to spot symptoms of a potential diabetic emergency. If you've been wondering whether certain herbs and nutritional supplements live up to their claims for treating diabetes, we shed light on that subject, too.

With diabetes, unlike so many other health concerns, your care doesn't revolve around a single, once-and-done decision: "Should I take that pill?" "Do I have surgery?" Instead, it entails a lifetime of choices: "What should I have for lunch?" "When can I work out today?" So in Part III, you'll find all kinds of strategies for shaping a diabetes-friendly lifestyle, from launching an exercise program to eating the right foods. You'll also get helpful advice on emotional matters, like coping with stress and depression. As studies have shown, your mood and mindset can have a dramatic impact on your ability to stay a step ahead of diabetes.

Because diet plays such an important role in treating diabetes, Part IV features a seven-day low-carbohydrate menu plan that's proven to rein in blood sugar and take off extra pounds. It's accompanied by a collection of more than two dozen recipes that deliver a healthy balance of smart carbs and beneficial fats. No diabetic diet ever tasted *this* good!

Make no mistake: Diabetes is a serious chronic

condition that requires a doctor's supervision and support. But thanks to modern medical advances, it's more manageable than ever. So seize this opportunity to take charge of your health. Because now more than ever, "living with diabetes" means living life your way.

PART I

Understanding Diabetes

CHAPTER ONE

The Big Picture

Although diabetes affects just 6.5 percent of the entire U.S. population, it ranks as the seventh leading cause of death in this country. Researchers estimate that by the year 2020, about 250 million people worldwide may be at significant risk for developing type 2 diabetes—the most common form of the disease, accounting for close to 95 percent of new cases.

But behind these grim statistics is some very good news. While we can't change certain risk factors for type 2 diabetes, like genetic makeup and age, we definitely can influence two of the big ones: weight and activity level. Eating healthfully and exercising regularly may not only help prevent diabetes but also minimize complications if we do get the disease.

JUST WHAT IS DIABETES?

Simply stated, diabetes is a breakdown in your body's ability to convert food into energy. Under normal conditions, your body relies on glucose, a type of sugar, to fuel its everyday functions. During the digestive process, your body extracts glucose from food and delivers it to hungry cells via the bloodstream, the body's main transportation system.

Of course, glucose has to get into each cell before it can serve as an energy source. This job falls to insulin, a hormone manufactured by the pancreas. You might think of insulin as the key that unlocks the door to let glucose into your cells. Usually, a problem with insulin sets the stage for diabetes.

Virtually everyone with diabetes experiences the same constellation of symptoms and faces the same potential complications. But doctors recognize three distinct forms of the disease: type 1, type 2, and gestational. Each plays out a bit differently in the body.

For example, in type 1 diabetes, the pancreas doesn't make enough insulin, explains Melissa D. Katz, M.D., assistant professor of medicine in the department of endocrinology and metabolism at Weill Medical College of Cornell University in New York City. Eventually, the pancreas shuts down production altogether. This is why everyone who has type 1 diabetes must take insulin. Because it typically occurs in childhood, type 1 diabetes sometimes is called juvenile diabetes.

In contrast, people who have type 2 diabetes are able to produce insulin, but not as much as their bodies need, Dr. Katz says. That's because they're insulin resistant. In other words, their bodies don't use insulin properly, which allows glucose to build up in the bloodstream instead of entering cells and getting converted into energy. The poor pancreas, caught in the crosshairs of this physiological misunderstanding, tries to correct the situation by pumping out even more insulin.

By itself, insulin resistance doesn't cause any obvious symptoms, other than an inability to lose weight. But if the pancreas can't keep up with the increased demand for insulin, insulin resistance eventually progresses to full-fledged type 2 diabetes. Still, not everyone who has type 2 needs to take insulin. Often this form of the disease responds well to lifestyle changes.

At one time, type 2 was known as adult-onset diabetes because it typically occurs after age 45. With the increasing number of overweight children in this country, however, doctors have reported an alarming surge in the number of young people with type 2.

The third form of diabetes, gestational diabetes, also involves insulin resistance. It's brought on by elevated insulin production during pregnancy—a result of the mom-to-be's weight gain, Dr. Katz says. Fortunately, gestational diabetes tends to subside once the baby arrives, though it can make a woman more likely to develop type 2 diabetes later in life. (We'll talk about this more in just a bit.)

WHO IS AT RISK?

While doctors don't yet know the exact cause of type 1 diabetes, it does have some identifiable risk factors, including genetics and ethnicity. For example, children whose parents are diabetic are more likely to develop type 1 diabetes. Likewise, whites are at higher risk for type 1 than blacks and Hispanics.

THE HISTORY OF INSULIN

Records of diabetes date back to ancient times. But no one had pinpointed insulin as the culprit until 1910, when a scientist named Sharpey-Shafer theorized that people with diabetes were missing a chemical in the pancreas. He called that chemical insulin. Another scientist, R. C. Paulesco, found that an extract from the pancreas effectively lowered blood sugar in dogs.

In 1922, a team of researchers at the University of Toronto went one step further. They actually removed the pancreases from dogs, so the animals developed diabetes. The researchers then extracted fluid from the islet cells of healthy dogs and injected it into the diabetic dogs. Their symptoms subsided. Later that year, the research team extracted pure insulin from the pancreas of a cow and gave it to a teenager with diabetes, whose symptoms improved dramatically.

The four scientists involved in the discovery were Frederick Banting, Charles Best, J. B. Collip, and J. J. R. Macleod. Banting and Macleod received the Nobel Prize for medicine in 1923, and they shared their prize money with the two other scientists. By then, insulin was widely available and had saved many lives.

Until 1978, most insulin came from animals, mainly cattle and pigs. But then researchers figured out how to manufacture insulin, making it the first human protein developed through biotechnology.

Even if you've inherited a predisposition to type 1 diabetes, the disease will kick in only in the presence of some other environmental factor, such as an illness. Most experts believe that certain viruses or autoimmune responses may be part of the triggering mechanism, Dr. Katz says.

As for type 2 diabetes, any of the following can raise your risk.

Ethnicity. According to Dr. Katz, insulin resistance seems to be more prevalent in certain ethnic groups. The incidence of type 2 diabetes is twice as high among blacks and Hispanics, and 6.3 percent higher among Native Americans, compared with whites.

Obesity. As with type 1 diabetes, any genetic tendency toward type 2 diabetes must be activated by an outside force, such as excess weight. Apple-shaped people, who have more upper-body fat, are more prone to insulin resistance, Dr. Katz says.

Age. Most cases of type 2 diabetes occur in people over age 45. So you should pay particularly close attention for any warning signs starting at midlife.

Previous bouts of gestational diabetes. "A woman who has had gestational diabetes during one or more of her pregnancies is at increased risk for developing type 2 diabetes later in life," Dr. Katz says. Your odds are even greater if one of your babies weighed nine or more pounds at birth.

Incidentally, the risk factors for gestational diabetes—which occurs in about 4 percent of all pregnancies—include obesity, a family history of maternal diabetes, and the occurrence of gestational diabetes in a previous pregnancy.

WHAT SHOULD I WATCH FOR?

With diabetes, the most recognizable symptoms result from fluid loss. After all, your body has to do something with the extra glucose that's floating around your bloodstream, unable to get into cells. Its solution is to eliminate the glucose in urine, which means

ASSESS YOUR DIABETES RISK

Many serious complications of diabetes can be avoided if the disease is diagnosed and treated early on. So at the first sign of symptoms, see your doctor without delay for a fasting plasma glucose test and a complete physical exam. Be aware, too, that you're at increased risk if you answer yes to even one of the following questions.

1. **Do you weigh more than you should?** The single greatest predictor of who gets type 2 diabetes and who doesn't is being overweight or obese. In fact, research by the Centers for Disease Control and Prevention (CDC) indicates that for every kilogram (2.2 pounds) of extra weight, the risk of diabetes climbs about 9 percent.
2. **Are you Hispanic, African American, or Native American?** Compared with the general population, people in these ethnic groups are twice as likely to develop type 2 diabetes.
3. **Do you seem to urinate more frequently than other people, even at night?** When you have too much glucose in your blood, your body attempts to remove the excess through urination. Over time, the extra workload can lead to kidney failure, requiring dialysis or even a kidney transplant.
4. **Are you thirsty all the time, no matter how much you drink?** Excessive glucose in your blood will suck up your body's stores of water. If you don't drink enough to replenish the supply, you may notice your skin drying out, too. Too much glucose can lead to a life-threatening state of dehydration called hyperglycemic hyperosmolar nonketotic syndrome (HHNS).
5. **Do you have an insatiable appetite?** In untreated diabetes, even though you're eating plenty, your cells may be starving from lack of fuel. They don't have insulin to deliver the glucose they need. This is why, besides being hungry, you might feel tired.
6. **Are you bothered by blurred vision?** When blood glucose climbs too high, it can affect the amount of water in the

lenses of your eyes. Over time, it can lead to retinopathy, a common—but preventable—cause of blindness.

7. **Do you frequently develop cramps in your legs, or tingling or numbness in your hands or feet?** These symptoms may signal the onset of the kind of nerve damage that can lead to permanent injury and even amputation.
8. **Do you have a history of gum, skin, bladder, or yeast infections?** Sugar provides ideal environmental conditions for bacterial growth, raising the risk of infection. In addition, excess sugar dulls immune function by handicapping white blood cells.
9. **Have you experienced recent sudden weight loss, in addition to severe fatigue, blurred vision, or other symptoms such as excessive urination or thirst?** These could be the first signs of type I diabetes. See your doctor or visit the emergency room without delay.

tapping into your body's water supply. This sets the stage for the following symptoms:

- Frequent urination
- Unusual thirst
- Unexplained weight loss
- Persistent fatigue for no apparent reason

You also may notice these warning signs:

- Slow healing of cuts and bruises
- Tingling or numbness in the hands and feet
- Recurring skin, gum, or bladder infections

Unfortunately, too many people overlook their symptoms until it's too late. By one estimate, for every two people who know they have diabetes, another is unaware of his or her illness. As many as six million Americans may be diabetic and not even realize it. With statistics like these, it becomes clear that the real problem with diabetes lies in missed or delayed diagnoses.

Collectively, the symptoms of diabetes are unmistakable. Individually, they could point to other ailments, notes Florence Brown, M.D., senior staff physician at the Joslin Diabetes Center at Harvard University. For example, sudden, unexplained weight loss may indicate an overactive thyroid gland. Excessive urination could suggest a urinary tract infection. And blurry vision, particularly after age 40, might be a byproduct of the aging process itself.

That's why everyone over age 45 should be tested for diabetes every three years, whether or not they notice any symptoms, advises Lynne M. Kirk, M.D., associate chief of the division of internal medicine at the University of Texas Southwestern Medical Center in Dallas. Likewise, if you have just one or two symptoms, you still should be checked for diabetes, particularly if you have any risk factors for the disease.

IS DIABETES PREVENTABLE?

A Finnish study found that many people can significantly lower their blood glucose levels—and their diabetes risk—simply by making appropriate lifestyle changes, such as eating a low-fat, high-fiber diet and getting regular exercise. So if you don't already have diabetes, here's some advice that could help sidestep the disease in the first place. (Already have diabetes? These strategies still make good sense for managing your blood sugar and avoiding complications.)

Take Off Those Extra Pounds

Research shows that people who have genes that increase their propensity for abdominal fat also carry genes that raise their risk of insulin resistance. In fact, a high proportion of abdominal fat to total body fat appears to induce insulin resistance.

You can get a better sense of your weight-related health risk by calculating your body mass index, or BMI. According to one study, people with BMIs of more than 27 may be insulin-resistant and at risk for diabetes. To figure out your BMI, first divide your weight in pounds by the square of your height in inches, then multiply that number by 705. Let's say you're 5-foot-5, or 65 inches, and 150 pounds. Your BMI would be 25, based on the following calculation: $65 \times 65 = 4225$; $150 \div 4225 = 0.036$; $0.036 \times 705 = 25$ (rounded off).

Incidentally, while slimming down may help protect against diabetes, developing the disease actually can inhibit weight loss. Doctors can't explain why, but they've noticed that those with diabetes have a harder time managing their weight than those without, says Diane Krieger, M.D., endocrinologist and director of the Diabetes Care Program in South Miami. Medication may be part of the problem; certain diabetes drugs seem to prompt the body to cling to extra pounds. The good news is, if you already have diabetes, dropping just 10 percent of your overall body weight can help stop the disease from progressing.

Launch an Exercise Program

When you engage in almost any form of physical activity, your muscles demand more glucose for fuel. As a result, your pancreas secretes more insulin. Exercise also enhances your body's ability to use insulin, so your cells are better able to convert glucose to energy.

If you've been relatively inactive, definitely consult your doctor before you begin working out. Then follow these guidelines to get the most from your exercise program.

Fit fitness into your daily routine. A half-hour of physical activity most days of the week can help prevent diabetes. And those thirty minutes don't need to be a grueling aerobic workout; a walk will do just as well. You can go for thirty minutes straight or divvy up the time into, say, three ten-minute sessions.

To maintain steady blood sugar levels, your best bet is to plan your workouts for about the same time every day. If you can't spare even ten minutes for exercise, find ways to incorporate more physical activity into your daily routine. Get up to change the channel on the TV rather than using the remote. Park your car and walk to the bank instead of using the drive-through window. Stand up and move around while you're on the phone, rather than sitting in a chair. These short bursts of activity add up!

Don't forget strength training. Lifting weights helps protect against diabetes by increasing the amount of glucose that's converted to energy. Ideally, you should plan for two or three strength-training sessions per week, with at least a day of rest between sessions.

Take precautions against blood sugar dips. You need to make sure your body has enough fuel for your workouts. If you plan to exercise more than an hour after a meal, eat a light carbohydrate snack beforehand. A more intense workout calls for a slightly heftier snack, like half of a meat sandwich or a cup of low-fat milk.

Stay a Step Ahead of Stress

When you're under stress, your body shifts into fight-or-flight mode. This prompts a host of physiological changes, including the release of extra glucose by the liver to provide fuel for your muscles. Any glucose that doesn't get into your cells floats around your bloodstream, potentially elevating your blood glucose level. Your pancreas responds by releasing more insulin—a reaction that, if triggered repeatedly over time, can contribute to diabetes risk.

Stress also may compromise your eating habits and your exercise program; when you're feeling tense and anxious, you're more likely to make poor food choices or skip workouts. That can elevate blood glucose levels, too.

Pay attention for signs of excessive stress, especially changes in your sleep pattern, energy level, appetite, or sex drive. If they persist, your best bet may be to seek help from a physician or counselor.

WHAT SHOULD I DO IF I THINK I HAVE DIABETES?

Your first step is to see your doctor for a proper diagnosis. He'll order a test to measure the amount of glucose in your blood. It's the only way to find out for certain whether you have diabetes. People with the disease will show above-normal glucose even if they haven't eaten for a while.

Normal blood glucose falls between 70 and 120. A reading in the low- to mid-100s indicates mild diabetes. In more severe cases, glucose can climb to between 200 and 300.

HOW DO DOCTORS TREAT DIABETES?

The goal of diabetes treatment is to keep blood glucose levels as close to normal as possible. For some people, lifestyle strategies—primarily a healthy diet and regular exercise—will be enough.

Actually, the "rules" for managing diabetes used to be much stricter. People were told that they couldn't eat sweets, couldn't play sports, and—as far as women were concerned—couldn't have babies. The disease limited their personal and professional choices and their freedom. Thank goodness all that has changed.

That's not to say living with diabetes is easy. It takes a lot of adjustment, especially in terms of your eating habits. To control your blood sugar, you need to follow a diet that pretty much dictates when and

THE TV–DIABETES LINK

For years, doctors have known that an active lifestyle protects against diabetes and all of its life-threatening complications. But researchers at the Harvard School of Public Health wanted to find out if the reverse also is true: Would long stretches of watching TV—the sedentary activity that consumes 40 percent of our leisure time—increase the odds of developing diabetes?

To find out, the researchers tracked the viewing habits of nearly 38,000 men, ages 40 to 75, for more than ten years. After adjusting for age, activity level, alcohol use, and smoking, the men who watched TV for more than four hours a day were more than twice as likely to develop diabetes as the men who watched TV for less than two hours a week. Those who spent forty hours a week glued to the tube tripled their risk.

And if you routinely stay up late to catch Leno or Letterman and then get up early the next morning, you may be even more vulnerable to diabetes. A study at the University of Chicago found that getting less than six-and-a-half hours of shut-eye a night raises the odds of insulin resistance, a diabetes precursor.

how much you eat. The guidelines tend to be a little more rigid with type 1, though good nutrition is very important to managing both type 1 and type 2.

Experts have found that people more easily adapt to long-term lifestyle changes when those changes make sense to them. So if you have diabetes, you should work with a nutritionist to help shape an eating plan that you feel good about and can live with. (We'll talk more about dietary strategies in Chapter 7.)

WHAT ABOUT MEDICATION?

Not everyone needs medication. For those who do, doctors likely will opt for one of the oral glucose-lowering drugs, called insulin sensitizers. These come in four classes, each of which has a unique action in the body.

- Sulfonylureas and meglitinides prompt the pancreas to secrete more insulin
- Thiazolidinediones make the body more sensitive to insulin
- Biguanides reduce the amount of sugar produced by the liver
- Alpha-glucosidase inhibitors delay the absorption of glucose

In choosing the best drug for a patient, doctors will take into account a variety of factors, including the person's symptoms as well as the drug's side effects. Many of the insulin sensitizers work in combination, notes James Rosenzweig, M.D., senior physician at the Joslin Diabetes Center in Boston. So if one particular drug doesn't produce the desired results, adding a second drug might do the trick.

In general, insulin injections are reserved for the most severe cases of diabetes. The insulin gets absorbed into the tissues underneath the skin, then circulates through the bloodstream. Injections into the stomach seem to work fast, while those into the upper arm or thigh take longer to produce effects. The type of insulin makes a difference, too: Some cause glucose to drop quickly, while others are mixed with a solution that slows their absorption.

CAN ALTERNATIVE MEDICINE HELP?

Certain herbs and nutritional supplements have shown promise not just to treat diabetes but also to prevent it. If you have diabetes, you shouldn't try these alternative therapies on your own. Instead, consult a naturopathic doctor (N.D.), who can monitor your response to treatment. And be sure to tell your other doctors about any herbs or supplements you're using. They can interfere with diabetes medications you're taking. (You'll learn more about the alternative medicine options in Chapter 4.)

WHAT ELSE SHOULD I KNOW ABOUT DIABETES CARE?

First, if you have diabetes, you must keep tabs on your blood glucose levels. Your doctor can help determine a target glucose range, which may vary slightly from the normal range. "Monitoring your blood sugar is a powerful tool," Dr. Brown notes. "It allows you to control your diabetes, rather than your diabetes controlling you." (For the latest on monitoring tools and technology, see Chapter 3.)

You need to stay on top of your blood fat levels, too. High cholesterol and high triglycerides can raise your risk of other serious health problems, including heart disease and stroke. Fortunately, blood fats respond to the same lifestyle strategies as blood sugar—namely, eating healthfully and exercising regularly.

Because you are more vulnerable to secondary health problems, you should consider scheduling regular checkups with appropriate specialists—a cardiologist for your heart, for example, or a nephrologist for your kidneys. "I recommend that all diabetes patients see an ophthalmologist twice a year, so any possible retinal disease is caught early," Dr. Katz says. Periodic visits to a podiatrist are helpful, too. A podiatrist can check for cuts and infections, which you may not notice because of decreased sensation in your feet—a common complication of diabetes.

IS A CURE FOR DIABETES WITHIN REACH?

For type 2 diabetes, the answer to this question can be found in lifestyle strategies, which in some cases can correct insulin resistance. For type 1, the outlook hasn't been quite as bright, because the insulin-producing islet cells in the pancreas are destroyed.

But the findings of a small pilot study offer new hope for those with type 1 diabetes. Researchers at the University of Alberta in Edmonton, Canada, discovered that with intravenous islet cell transplants, study participants began producing their own insulin, which meant they could stop their daily insulin injections. Two years after the study, six of the seven participants still did not need injections.

Since then, another thirty-two people have received experimental islet cell transplants at ten medical centers in the United States, Canada, and Europe. If the procedure proves successful, experts expect that it will become a routine treatment for type 1 diabetes.

IF I HAVE DIABETES, HOW CAN I IMPROVE MY PROGNOSIS?

As with any chronic illness, managing diabetes presents its share of physical and psychological challenges. Your long-term health depends on your ability to make lifestyle choices that will keep the disease in check. To maintain the right mindset for this full-time job, experts offer these suggestions. (For more, turn to Chapter 5.)

Accept your condition. When first diagnosed with diabetes, most people go through a denial phase. That's perfectly normal. But it can be a problem if it persists, because you may not be as vigilant about your self-care as you should. If you frequently cheat on your eating plan, for example, or you routinely skip your blood sugar tests, you could jeopardize your health in the long run. To get back on track, try writing down what you do for self-care and why each step is so important.

Blow off some steam. The stress of managing diabetes can feel overwhelming. But don't let it get the best of you. Joining a diabetes support group could help. So could engaging in relaxing, rewarding activities. Sign up for dance lessons or pottery classes, volunteer for a charity, take up tai chi or yoga—whatever brings you pleasure and peace.

Never give up. Remember, your blood sugar level responds to factors other than lifestyle choices, like illness and major life events. So if you experience an unexpected blood sugar spike, don't abandon your self-care. Just stay the course, and eventually your blood sugar should return to normal. Of course, if it remains high, you should see your doctor.

CHAPTER TWO

The Hidden Risks

It's relatively common knowledge that diabetes is a serious chronic disease. Which makes this bit of information even more astonishing: According to some estimates, only one-third of those with type 2 diabetes take their medication regularly. Without it, they run the risk of uncontrolled high blood sugar, which could lead to even more serious health problems in the future.

Of course, effectively managing diabetes isn't only about taking medication. It also involves making smart food choices, increasing physical activity, and keeping tabs on blood sugar levels. Yes, it's a lot of work. But it's much better than the alternative.

You see, by not being vigilant about your diabetes care, you're gambling on whether you'll develop the sorts of complications that all too frequently occur ten to fifteen years down the road. "If you let your blood sugar chronically go into the 200 range without doing anything about it, you could experience serious problems later on, even though you might feel perfectly fine now," explains James Rosenzweig, M.D., senior

GO TO THE PROS

If you feel you need more support and supervision to manage diabetes and prevent its complications, consider paying a visit to one of the many diabetes centers throughout the country. Often they're affiliated with teaching hospitals. You'll work with a team of professionals—a diabetes educator, a nutritionist, and possibly an exercise physiologist, in addition to a primary care physician or endocrinologist—to develop a self-care plan that meets your unique needs. The centers also provide access to specialists in cardiology, optometry, and podiatry, who can work with the rest of your team to address any complications you may be experiencing.

physician at the Joslin Diabetes Center in Boston. These problems include heart and kidney disease, as well as blindness and amputation resulting from damage to the circulatory and nervous systems.

HEART DISEASE: DIABETES' DANGEROUS COMPANION

If you have diabetes, you need to be concerned about heart disease. In fact, you're more likely to develop heart disease than a smoker who has no other risk factors. If that isn't eye-opening enough, consider this: Two-thirds of people with diabetes will die from some form of heart or blood vessel disease.

The good news is, many of the lifestyle strategies that help control diabetes also will help fight heart disease. Slimming down to a healthy weight, eating a low-fat, high-fiber diet, and improving physical fitness all can lead to better blood sugar and a stronger heart.

Stabilizing your blood sugar levels may improve your measures for the four heart health markers on page 25.

Beyond basic lifestyle improvements, experts recommend the following to reduce heart disease risk.

Know your cholesterol profile. The standard advice is to keep total cholesterol below 200—and the lower, the better, especially if you have diabetes. High cholesterol can make arteries narrower, less flexible, and less likely to dilate properly during exercise or at other times when the heart needs more blood. High cholesterol also produces fatty deposits, or plaques, on artery walls. If a plaque should rupture—which is even more likely when high blood pressure is a factor—it can block an artery. As many as 80 percent of heart attacks result from ruptured plaques.

If you smoke, quit. Quitting is hard, but it can make a real difference in terms of your heart health. Every time you smoke, your blood pressure shoots upward, staying high for an hour or more. So if you light up even ten times a day, your blood pressure may constantly hover in the danger zone.

What's more, smoking negatively affects the ratio of good fats and bad fats in your blood. Specifically, it reduces levels of beneficial high-density lipoproteins (HDL) while raising levels of artery-clogging low-density lipoproteins (LDL). And it damages the structure of the LDL molecules, making them even more likely to stick to artery walls.

Try a new margarine. Traditional margarine contains hydrogenated fats, which can raise cholesterol as much as saturated fats. Some new brands of margarine—such as Benecol and Take Control—contain plant sterols, compounds that help prevent cholesterol from getting into the blood. One large study found that people who used Benecol for one year experienced a drop in total cholesterol of 10 percent and a decrease in LDL of 14 percent. According to other data, even people who are on medication can get an additional 15 percent reduction in LDL by consuming two servings of this heart-friendly margarine every day.

Manage stress better. Emotional stress can temporarily spike blood pressure and trigger heart attacks in people who have underlying cardiovascular problems. So experts recommend making a conscious effort to relax—whether through meditation, deep breathing, exercise, or some other activity.

"In real life, completely eliminating stress is hard," says Howard Weitz, M.D., co-director of the Jefferson Heart Institute of Thomas Jefferson University Hospital in Philadelphia. "Often people need professional counseling or a technique such as biofeedback to get adequate results." (For more helpful ideas on how to rein in stress, see Chapter 5.)

KIDNEY DISEASE: SYMPTOMLESS BUT SERIOUS

At least 40 million Americans either have kidney disease or are at high risk for it. And many of them are diabetics, according to a new analysis of government statistics conducted by the National Kidney Foundation.

The kidneys are delicate organs that contain millions of tiny blood vessels with even tinier molecule-

HEART HEALTH BY THE NUMBERS

If you have diabetes, you're two to four times more likely to suffer a heart attack than someone who doesn't. This is why you need to be especially vigilant about your heart health. Talk with your doctor about scheduling regular screenings to monitor the most common heart disease markers. In general, you're in great shape if you meet these goals:

- Triglycerides (a type of blood fat): below 200 milligrams/deciliter (mg/dl)
- LDL cholesterol: below 100 mg/dl
- HDL: above 47 mg/dl
- Blood pressure: below 135/85 mm Hg

size holes that essentially act as filters for the entire body. Under normal circumstances, digestive waste products squeeze through the tiny holes en route to their eventual elimination as urine. Useful substances, such as protein and red blood cells, are too big to pass through the holes, so they stay in the blood.

Diabetes can do serious damage to this sensitive system. When blood sugar levels are high, the kidneys must process more blood, which places extra stress on the filtering mechanism. If the kidneys operate on overload for too long, they eventually may start to leak. Useful protein molecules are able to pass through the filters, so they're lost in the urine, leading to a condition known as microalbuminuria.

Complicating this scenario is high blood pressure, which often occurs in tandem with uncontrolled diabetes. The higher the blood pressure, the more blood that is forced through the kidneys' fragile filters.

The kidneys' remarkable ability to continue working hard even under tremendous stress helps explain why they show few signs of trouble until they've lost almost all of their function. And the symptoms that do appear are rather vague—fluid buildup at first, possibly followed by loss of sleep, poor appetite, upset stomach, weakness, and difficulty concentrating.

To catch kidney problems as early as possible, you should schedule an annual blood pressure screening, along with a blood test for creatinine (to determine whether the kidneys are filtering the right waste products), and a urine check for protein (indicating the wrong waste products). Ask your doctor to use an albumin-specific dipstick test or to send your urine sample to a lab for analysis. Either one can identify even low levels of protein in your urine.

Fortunately, you can lower your risk of diabetic kidney disease just by keeping your blood sugar within your target range. Research has shown that maintaining tight control of blood sugar can reduce the likelihood of even small amounts of protein appearing in the urine by one-third. Those who have already tested positive for small amounts of protein can cut their risk of developing full-blown kidney disease by half. Other studies have suggested that maintaining healthy blood sugar can reverse microalbuminuria.

HIGH BLOOD PRESSURE: DASH TO THE RESCUE

If you're concerned about diabetes-related kidney trouble, you need to pay attention to your blood pressure as well as your blood sugar. You'll help protect your kidneys—and as a bonus, you'll lower your risk of heart disease.

Among the best strategies for lowering your blood pressure are losing weight and engaging in regular physical activity. But you also may be wondering whether you need to redefine your relationship with salt—long implicated as a contributor to blood pressure trouble.

The relationship between sodium and high blood pressure has generated quite a bit of controversy. Doctors have known for years that people who are "sodium-sensitive" experience spikes in their blood pressure readings when they get too much salt in their diets. But what about the rest of us?

According to the latest thinking, nearly everyone may benefit from reducing their salt intake. Sodium attracts water, so too much salt dramatically increases your blood volume—much of which is water to begin with. This, in turn, raises blood pressure.

The American Heart Association recommends that everyone limit their salt consumption to no more than 2,400 milligrams a day. You can start by switching to low-sodium or sodium-free processed foods and avoiding pickles, sauerkraut, and other salty foods.

If you're not ready to give up your saltshaker, experts suggest that you add salt at the table, not at the stove. The reason: Foods absorb a lot of salt during cooking, which reduces the intensity of their natural flavors. This means you need to sprinkle on even more salt to satisfy your taste buds. By adding salt at the table instead, you get the most flavor from the smallest amount.

Also, remember to read food labels. Sodium hides in some unexpected places. Even healthful whole-grain breakfast cereals may contain more than 100 milligrams of sodium per serving. Snack foods are in a class by themselves: An eight-ounce bag of potato chips may contain 1,300 milligrams of sodium, more than 50 percent of the recommended daily limit. By using the nutrition information on labels to keep a running tally of the sodium in foods, you're less likely to overdo.

If you prefer a more structured eating plan to help manage your blood pressure, you may want to try DASH, short for Dietary Approaches to Stop Hypertension. DASH is among the best strategies for treating and preventing high blood pressure. The diet calls for eight to ten daily servings of fruits and vegetables, seven or eight daily servings of whole grains, two or three daily servings of low-fat dairy foods, and no more than two daily servings of meat.

Many people who follow DASH are able to lower their systolic pressure (the top number in a blood pressure reading) by more than 11 points and their diastolic pressure (the bottom number) by more than 5 points. These results are as good as some would get from medication.

RETINOPATHY: SET YOUR SIGHTS ON PREVENTION

Almost everyone who has diabetes shows some signs of an eye disease called retinopathy. Each year, as many as 24,000 of them lose their eyesight to the disease.

Retinopathy occurs when microscopic blood clots form inside the light-sensitive tissues of the eyes. New research shows that taking a low-dose aspirin every day—the same recommendation to help diabetics reduce their risk of heart attack—may help prevent diabetes-related vision trouble as well.

Researchers at Harvard University's Schepens Eye Research Institute discovered that long before people with diabetes notice any vision changes, they have tiny clots blocking blood flow inside their eyes. The researchers further determined that the clots contain platelets, which normally play a role in blood coagulation, and fibrin, which is a protein. Both substances contribute to the clots that lead to heart attacks.

While the study did not test whether a daily low-dose aspirin could reduce clotting in the eyes, researcher Mara Lorenzi, M.D., recommends starting aspirin therapy as soon as possible after getting a diabetes diagnosis—with your doctor's approval, of course. The aspirin should help, since it's known to interfere with the formation of clots, Dr. Lorenzi says.

Another advance in the fight against diabetes-related vision damage has to do with the guidelines for eye exams. Until recently, experts have advised people with type 1 diabetes to get an exam within three to five years of their diabetes diagnoses. But now some say that type 1 diabetics should be scheduled for a special retinal exam within 1 year of diagnosis. The reason: A study involving more than 1,600 people with type 1 found that 67 percent developed retinopathy within five years of finding out they have diabetes.

In the exam, the doctor administers eyedrops to dilate the pupils, then checks the blood vessels in the retina for signs of trouble. Some experts believe that people with type 2 diabetes should get this screening every year as well.

PERIPHERAL NEUROPATHY: PROPER FOOT CARE IS KEY

Another common diabetes complication is peripheral neuropathy, in which uncontrolled high blood sugar damages nerve cells, causing a loss of sensation. Because the nerves in the feet are the longest in the body, the feet usually suffer most, becoming vulnerable to injury and sores. Sores that don't heal properly can become ulcerated and infected; the most serious ones can lead to amputation. An estimated six in 1,000 people with diabetes lose a limb to amputation.

What's saddest about this statistic is that the vast majority of those procedures could be avoided. If you have diabetes, your feet need a little extra TLC. Here's what experts recommend.

Make an appointment with a foot specialist. From the moment you find out you have diabetes, you should see a podiatrist on a regular basis, says Marc A. Brenner, D.P.M., director of the Institute of Diabetic Foot Research in Glendale, New York. This foot specialist can determine whether you have neuropathy and help take care of your feet if you do. For example, trimming toenails and treating calluses and corns can be dangerous for people with neuropathy and should be done by a podiatric professional.

Wear quality socks. The best are made from a combination of cotton and synthetic material. On very cold days, slip on two pairs—a thin one next to your skin, followed by a thicker one. "The more insulation between your foot and the ground, the better," Dr. Brenner notes.

Make sure the shoe fits. Your shoe size should be determined by a certified pedorthist, a person who's specially trained to measure feet, Dr. Brenner says. Ask your podiatrist to recommend a shoe store that offers such services. Do your shoe shopping in the afternoon, when your feet are more likely to be swollen.

Wrap your feet in sneaks. You probably won't need to get custom shoes. A high-quality cross-training or running shoe should serve just as well. Look for a pair with a roomy toebox; a removable inlay to fit in a custom orthotic device; a thick, padded tongue; and cushioning for the ball and heel of the foot.

Wear an orthotic. A diabetic orthotic is a custom-made device that fits into your shoe. It reduces pressure in certain spots, or spreads pressure across the entire foot. Your podiatrist can help assess your need for an orthotic and measure you for one, if appropriate.

Do a daily inspection. Check for any discoloration, swelling, or sores, using a large mirror to see each foot from all angles. Better yet, ask someone to check for you. Be sure the person touches your feet; if either one feels hot, it could signal an infection.

Take those dogs swimming. Even if you have neuropathy, you still need to exercise. Swimming is safest, Dr. Brenner says, because you don't put any pressure on your feet. When you get out of the pool, carefully dry your feet and sprinkle them with foot powder to prevent fungal and yeast infections.

GUM DISEASE: NOTHING TO SMILE ABOUT

While scientists don't fully understand the relationship between gum disease and diabetes, they do know that gum disease may threaten more than your smile. For starters, it appears to trigger the clinical onset of diabetes in people who are predisposed to the disease. Furthermore, it may undermine a person's ability to effectively manage diabetes.

When researchers analyzed data from the Third National Health and Nutrition Examination Survey, they found that among overweight adults with the highest insulin resistance levels, one in two also suffered from severe gum disease. It's possible that gum disease, which results from chronic bacterial infection involving the entire body, somehow provokes insulin resistance. The process may have a connection to the inflammatory substances produced in response to infection. Molecules of these substances prevent insulin from docking in its receptors on the surface of cells. This reduces the uptake of glucose by the cells, leading to insulin resistance.

"Oral health is far more important than we previously thought," acknowledges Sara G. Grossi, D.D.S., assistant professor of oral biology at the School of Dental Medicine at State University of New York at Buffalo and director of the university's Periodontal

SYNDROME X: NO LONGER A MYSTERY

You may know syndrome X by its other name: metabolic syndrome. It's a cluster of symptoms—such as obesity, high blood pressure, hyperlipidemia (elevated blood fat levels), and high insulin levels—that together raise heart disease risk.

People with syndrome X also test positive for insulin resistance, in which the body has a difficult time converting glucose to energy. The pancreas churns out plenty of insulin, but the hormone can't seem to get glucose into cells. So, much of the glucose just floats around in the bloodstream.

This is why people with syndrome X typically have blood glucose levels at the upper end of the normal range. Still, they may not develop full-blown diabetes. Many people with syndrome X don't.

Syndrome X has a very strong link to obesity. In fact, being overweight is one of its most common signs. Extra body fat lowers your sensitivity to insulin and raises your risk for heart disease.

Not surprisingly, the standard treatment for syndrome X includes losing weight—even if only ten or fifteen pounds—and increasing physical activity. Exercise does more than melt away those extra pounds; it also enhances insulin sensitivity and lowers blood pressure. In those cases requiring medication, doctors usually prescribe statins, which help reduce blood fat levels.

Disease Research Center. "Gum disease may impact other conditions, such as heart disease, stroke, respiratory problems, and diabetes. It constitutes a significant health risk for people with diabetes, since it could lead to difficulty controlling blood sugar and therefore worsen diabetic status."

Your best bet for preventing gum disease is to brush and floss your teeth at least twice each day, eat

POLYCYSTIC OVARY SYNDROME: WOMEN, BE WARY

An alarming number of American women—an estimated 6 to 10 percent—have polycystic ovary syndrome (PCOS). Many don't even know it. It's the most common endocrine condition in premenopausal women and the leading cause of infertility in the United States.

Many women with PCOS are insulin resistant or glucose intolerant (meaning they have excess insulin in their blood). As a result, they're more likely to become diabetic than the general population. In fact, one in ten women with PCOS develops diabetes by age 40.

Some of that extra insulin finds its way to the ovaries, where it attaches to receptors and directs the ovaries to increase their production of testosterone. In the liver, the insulin interacts with sex hormones, also helping to raise the level of testosterone. This is why women with PCOS are prone to facial hair and acne. They may experience irregular menstrual periods, or they may not ovulate at all.

PCOS often develops at puberty, but many women remain undiagnosed until they're in their twenties or thirties. Screening for the condition involves a physical exam and blood tests to rule out other health problems.

As far as treatment, hormones and medication can take care of facial hair and acne. If you're not trying to get pregnant, your doctor probably will prescribe oral contraceptives to regulate your periods. If you are trying to get pregnant, you'll need hormones to help ovulate and conceive.

a balanced diet rich in antioxidants, and schedule regular appointments for dental exams and teeth cleanings. Your dentist will tell you how often he wants to see you.

PART II

The Best in Diabetes Self-Care

CHAPTER THREE

Breakthroughs in Blood Sugar Control

Chronically high blood sugar can take a tremendous toll on the body, affecting the heart, kidneys, nerves, and eyes. Every year, at least 190,000 people die from diabetes and its various complications.

"Don't let the statistics scare you, though," says Anne Daly, R.D., C.D.E., a certified diabetes educator and president of health care and education for the American Diabetes Association in Springfield, Illinois. "The people reflected in these numbers didn't have access to the tools and techniques now available for managing blood sugar."

THE REWARDS OF TIGHT CONTROL

A wealth of research about diabetes underscores the value of taking good care of yourself. First and foremost, that means keeping your blood sugar as close to normal as possible—what experts describe as tight control.

One particular study, the Diabetes Control and Complications Trial (DCCT), divided 1,441 people with type 1 diabetes into two groups. One took a highly aggressive approach to treatment, aiming for tight control. The other followed a more conventional protocol, doing just enough to avoid any overt symptoms of high or low blood sugar. After six-and-a-half years, the group aiming for tight control had reduced kidney disease by 56 percent, nerve damage by 57 percent, vision problems by 76 percent, and certain heart conditions, like atherosclerosis, by 41 percent. Based on these findings, intensive therapy can effectively delay the onset and slow the progression of diabetes complications.

In the United Kingdom Prospective Diabetes Study (UKPDS), people with type 2 diabetes experienced similar benefits from tight control. In fact, for every percentage point of improvement in blood glucose levels—based on tests over three months—the overall risk of complications dropped by 35 percent.

"The reward of tight control is directly related to one's commitment to keeping blood sugar in the normal range from hour to hour, day in and day out," concludes Lois Jovanovic, M.D., an endocrinologist who specializes in diabetes in women.

TESTS: YOUR MOST IMPORTANT TASK

To effectively manage your blood sugar, you must check it on a regular basis. Of course, what's "regular" for you might not be for someone else. You and your doctor should work together to identify the basic pattern in the rise and fall of your blood sugar levels.

FIVE MUST-HAVE TESTS

If you've been diagnosed with diabetes, your doctor likely will recommend the following tests as part of your self-care plan (and if he doesn't, be sure to ask). They're essential to effectively controlling your condition and heading off potential complications.

Test	Frequency
Blood sugar screening, self-administered	Daily
Blood test for glycosylated hemoglobin	At least once a year
Foot check for sores or ulcers, performed by a podiatrist	At least once a year
Eye screening for retinopathy	Once a year
Lipid panel, including total cholesterol, HDL, LDL, and triglycerides	Once a year

Then you can adjust the frequency of your testing accordingly.

For example, if your blood sugar pretty much stays where it ought to be, your doctor may decide that you can cut back on your tests to just three days a week. More changeable blood sugar may require monitoring every day, or even more than once a day.

Keep in mind that you might need to adjust your testing schedule on occasion, depending on what's going on in your life. Illness and stress can raise your blood sugar, as can overeating. So you should step up your testing then, especially if you experience any symptoms of high blood sugar. They include headache, blurred vision, intense thirst, frequent urination, and dry, itchy skin.

On the other hand, if you feel shaky, nervous, confused, tired, or hungry, your blood sugar may have dropped too low. It can happen when you don't eat enough, or you exercise too hard or too long, or you take a bit too much diabetes medication. You'll feel better if you consume a small amount of a simple carbohydrate, like half a cup of a regular (non-diet) soft drink or fruit juice, a few hard candies, or a tablespoon of sugar. And be sure to check your blood sugar, too.

HOW TO MAKE THE MOST OF MONITORING

Understanding how various factors influence your blood sugar can make a world of difference in how you manage your diabetes. To get maximum benefit from your tests, experts offer these tips.

Establish a schedule. If you haven't already done it, you should check your blood sugar four times a day for several weeks, advises Carla Miller, Ph.D., R.D., co-director of the Diet Assessment Center at Pennsylvania State University in University Park. This helps establish a baseline for your blood sugar readings, which you and your doctor can use to set up your monitoring schedule, as mentioned above. Do the test first thing in the morning, one to two hours after lunch and dinner, and right before bed.

Assess the impact of dietary changes. When making any sort of adjustments in your eating habits, be sure to check your blood sugar right before each meal and again two hours after. Your readings should be between 90 and 130 milligrams per deciliter (mg/

dl) prior to eating. Postmeal, they should not exceed 160.

Be watchful during workouts. As with dietary changes, you need to keep close tabs on your blood sugar when launching a new exercise program. Ideally, you should check it right before and right after each workout, says Robert Hanisch, senior medical exercise physiologist and certified diabetes educator for the Diabetes Treatment Center at Columbia–St. Mary's Hospital in Milwaukee. If your blood sugar is low—between 100 and 120 mg/dl—beforehand, eat a piece of fruit or drink half a cup of juice. Each has about 15 grams of carbohydrate, which can elevate blood sugar about 25 points. Do the same if your blood sugar drops after exercise.

Do spot checks. Most people with diabetes check their blood sugar once a day, usually first thing in the morning. Dr. Miller recommends an occasional test after lunch or in the evening, so you get a more complete picture of what influences your blood sugar level. Incidentally, the average blood sugar reading is between 110 and 150 at bedtime.

Take notes. Keep a written record of your blood sugar readings, along with what and when you ate, and when and for how long you exercised. "Use a spiral-bound notebook, or make up a spreadsheet on your computer," Dr. Miller suggests. Share your notes with your doctor. The information you collect can help determine whether you need to modify your self-care.

Try the latest tools. Scientists constantly are coming up with new gadgets to improve the accuracy and ease of blood sugar testing. You may want to ask your doctor about the following:

Continuous glucose sensor monitor. Available since 2000, this device measures blood sugar every twenty seconds, averages it every five minutes, and stores the information for three days straight. This allows for more precise monitoring than a few pricks of the skin throughout the day. The sensor is inserted in tissue just under the skin, and the monitor—about the size of a beeper—can be worn almost anywhere.

"It's a breakthrough in preventing hypoglycemia and hyperglycemia," says Frank Schwartz, M.D., clinical associate professor of medicine, endocrinology, and metabolism at West Virginia University School of Medicine in Parkersburg. "Among other benefits, it may reduce the incidence of car accidents involving people who didn't know they had hypoglycemia, or low blood sugar, and passed out at the wheel." (For more information on these conditions, see "Symptoms You Should Never Ignore" on the opposite page.)

Glycosylated hemoglobin test. Also known as HbA1c, this test evaluates how well you're managing your blood glucose over the long term by providing a percentage of average blood sugar concentration for a ninety-day period. "Schedule the test every three months, so you can make necessary changes before high blood glucose takes a toll," advises Dr. Jovanovic, who also is director and chief scientific officer at Sansum Medical Research Institute in Santa Barbara, California, and clinical professor of medicine at the University of Southern California, Los Angeles.

SYMPTOMS YOU SHOULD NEVER IGNORE

Because diabetes is a serious condition, even when it's kept under tight control, you should consult your doctor before making any changes in your eating or exercise habits. What's more, you must pay attention for early signs of three common diabetes complications that require prompt medical attention: severe hyperglycemia, hypoglycemia, and ketoacidosis.

Hyperglycemia occurs when your blood sugar level spikes too high. Its symptoms include increased thirst, frequent urination, fatigue, and unexplained weight loss. If your blood sugar stays elevated, despite your efforts to rein it in, you need to see your doctor as soon as possible, advises Christopher D. Saudek, M.D., director of the Johns Hopkins Diabetes Center in Baltimore.

In hypoglycemia, blood sugar drops too low, causing shakiness, dizziness, confusion, headache, sudden mood changes, and a tingling sensation around the mouth. Most people can treat mild hypoglycemia on their own by taking three glucose tablets, eating five or six pieces of hard candy, or drinking half a cup of fruit juice. The trick is, you must intervene quickly. If your blood sugar continues to decline, you could pass out. In addition, while hypoglycemia is common among diabetics, be sure to tell your doctor if your bouts are especially frequent or your symptoms quite severe.

Ketoacidosis affects only those with type I diabetes. It's a serious, potentially life-threatening condition in which blood levels of acids called ketones become dangerously high, poisoning the body. Its symptoms include increased thirst, frequent urination, nausea, vomiting, and fatigue. If you suspect you may have ketoacidosis, call your doctor or emergency medical number immediately.

A WAKE-UP CALL TO NIGHTTIME BLOOD SUGAR DIPS

All of us have a metabolic mechanism that triggers the gradual release of growth hormone and cortisol starting at around 4:00 A.M., so we have the get-up-and-go to roll out of bed when the alarm goes off. But some people get a more potent burst of these wake-up hormones than others. Since the hormones also suppress insulin production, a "morning person" who has diabetes might wake up to blood sugar of more than 240 mg/dl. This pattern is known as the dawn phenomenon, Dr. Jovanovic explains.

The quick fix for the dawn phenomenon is to take a larger dose of insulin that day. But you really should try to avoid high blood sugar to begin with. One solution to discuss with your doctor is to bump your long-acting dose from before dinner—the usual timing—to before bed. Then it would better match the release of wake-up hormones.

If, despite changes to your insulin protocol, you still can't prevent the dawn phenomenon, you could be a prime candidate for an insulin pump. This battery-operated device administers insulin through a tube, to help maintain consistent blood sugar levels. "Insulin pumps aren't the big black boxes they used to be," notes Dr. Jovanovic, who sports one herself. "Today's models could be mistaken for a pager that you clip on your belt or hide under your clothes." They can be programmed to deliver a small amount of insulin for the first half of the night and a larger

NOW AVAILABLE: NEEDLE-FREE INSULIN INJECTIONS

Need insulin, but can't tolerate the shots? Then you'll appreciate one of the latest advances in diabetes management: the jet injector. This device actually sprays insulin under your skin, which helps make frequent doses much more bearable. Jet injectors are available through a variety of manufacturers. Ask your doctor for a prescription.

amount for the rest of the night, she adds.

Regardless of your morning blood sugar level, experts recommend checking it around 3:00 A.M. for a few nights. This may seem impractical, but it can help determine whether you're prone to nighttime hypoglycemia. With this condition, you'll get an even bigger burst of wake-up hormones to help compensate for the shortfall in blood sugar.

You may be able to control nighttime hypoglycemia by eating fewer carbohydrates at your evening meals. This in turn could curb the release of growth hormone and cortisol, preventing the dawn phenomenon, Dr. Jovanovic says.

SPECIAL CARE FOR MOMS-TO-BE

For women who have diabetes, the prospect of pregnancy can raise all kinds of questions and concerns, especially with regard to blood sugar control. But they don't need to abandon their dreams of motherhood. With a little extra care, they can deliver perfectly healthy babies.

Even the conventional wisdom that women who have type 1 diabetes should not become pregnant no longer applies. "By adhering to the principles of tight control, a type 1 diabetic has the same chances of a normal pregnancy as a nondiabetic," Dr. Jovanovic says. "As long as the woman passes certain tests, I'll give her clearance to get pregnant." Specifically, Dr. Jovanovic looks for the following:

- Normal HbA1c tests
- Normal blood pressure
- Normal kidney function
- Stable eye status
- Normal gynecological exam

For women with type 2 diabetes, the treatment protocol is virtually the same as for gestational or pregnancy-induced diabetes. During pregnancy, both type 1 and type 2 diabetics must set strict mealtimes and be extra-vigilant about counting carbohydrates.

"And if they haven't been testing their blood sugar levels five to ten times a day, they will be," Dr. Jovanovic says. "My guidelines for a diabetic mom-to-be are even stricter than for the general public. She must keep her blood sugar at the absolute lowest end of the normal range without getting hypoglycemia. That's between 55 and 70 mg/dl premeal and below 140 mg/dl one hour postmeal."

Maintaining blood sugar at the lowest healthy level helps reduce the risk of birth defects. It also diminishes the likelihood of delivering a high-birth-weight

REZULIN: THE RISE AND FALL OF A DIABETES DRUG

Depending on how long you've had diabetes, you may recall the controversy surrounding Rezulin, which debuted in March 1997 as one of the most promising oral medications ever marketed for treating type 2 diabetes. Designed for use in conjunction with insulin or sulfonylureas, it lowered blood sugar by improving insulin sensitivity.

Rezulin showed so much potential that it moved to the fast track for FDA approval, avoiding much of the red tape involved in earning the agency's green light. By December 1997, some 600,000 Americans were taking the drug.

Then the FDA began receiving reports that about 2 percent of Rezulin users showed mildly elevated liver enzymes, suggesting liver irritation. In response, the agency advised everyone on the medication to schedule liver function tests every three months, and to stop taking Rezulin if they showed any signs of liver trouble.

In early 1998, the FDA learned that 150 more Americans had developed liver problems while on Rezulin, and that three people in Japan had died. The agency stepped up its testing guidelines, requiring liver tests *before* starting the drug, plus every month for six months *after* starting the drug and every two months for the rest of the first year. Rezulin's manufacturer, Warner-Lambert, revised the medication's label several times to include warnings for liver damage.

But with continued reports of liver damage and deaths, consumer groups lobbied fiercely against Rezulin. On March 21, 2000, the FDA asked Warner-Lambert to pull the drug from the market. The good news: Two other drugs, Avandia and Actos, work just as well and are safer for the liver.

baby, which can happen when too much sugar passes into the placenta.

Blood-sugar spikes exceeding 140 mg/dl are the leading cause of birth defects in babies born to women with diabetes. So if you become hypoglycemic, be careful not to overcompensate. The worst-case scenario is that you'd become unconscious and you'd be given an injection that sends your blood sugar soaring from 20 to 600 mg/dl, Dr. Jovanovic says.

If you're diabetic and pregnant, you must have a plan for your care in the event that you black out. Tell those most likely to be with you—family, friends, and co-workers—that you should be given only half of your normal injection amount. If you're still unconscious after ten minutes, you can be given the rest of the injection. If you remain unresponsive, then the person caring for you should call for help. That person also will need to inform the emergency medical technicians that you're pregnant and that you've already been given an injection.

What about breastfeeding? It's fine, even if you're insulin-dependent. The insulin won't affect your baby. As always, you will need to monitor your blood sugar, so you don't develop hypoglycemia. Since your baby will take in more of your glucose as he grows, your insulin requirements will gradually decrease over time.

CHAPTER FOUR

News from the Natural Arsenal

Natural medicine is not a passing fad. Experts estimate that roughly 80 percent of the global population relies on herbs for health care. In France, 30 to 40 percent of doctors use mostly botanical medicines in their practices. And in neighboring Germany, seven of every ten doctors prescribe herbal remedies to their patients.

In fact, the German people have so embraced herbs for their therapeutic value that the German government has appointed an expert panel to review herbal medicines for their safety and effectiveness. The panel, called Commission E, is a veritable who's who of Germany's physicians, pharmacologists, and herb specialists. Here in the United States, herb practitioners increasingly depend on Commission E reports, as well as other key research, for reliable evaluations of an herb's healing action and possible side effects.

Of course, for diabetes, the combination of a healthy diet and regular exercise—accompanied by medication, when necessary—remains the first and best choice for treatment. But certain herbs and nutritional supplements may provide extra support for stabilizing blood sugar levels. Some also have therapeutic properties that could prevent the onset of complications.

With a serious, chronic condition like diabetes, you should never try any alternative therapy—even a natural remedy like an herb or a nutritional supplement—on your own. Instead, discuss your options with your doctor. Since he's familiar with your situation, he can offer advice on what to try and what to watch for, in terms of an adverse reaction. If your doctor doesn't mention it, be sure to bring up any medication that you're taking. Conventional pharmaceuticals and natural therapies don't always mix.

This isn't intended to dissuade you from trying herbs and nutritional supplements. On the contrary, they can be a valuable component of your self-care plan. You just need to learn how to use them for maximum benefit. The same rule applies for any medication.

Of all the available herbs and nutritional supplements, the following nine have shown the most promise as diabetes treatments. Your doctor can help decide which might be best for you.

ALPHA-LIPOIC ACID: THE FIRST CHOICE TO FIGHT NERVE DAMAGE

The human body makes its own supply of alpha-lipoic acid, a little-known antioxidant. But production seems to slow down over time. Some experts believe that the decline in alpha-lipoic acid may be responsible for many of the health problems usually associated with aging.

Studies prove that alpha-lipoic acid prevents free radical damage to your cells, in part by recycling vitamins C and E. Because of this property, it may be useful against everything from aging and heart disease to Parkinson's disease and lupus. Scientists need to do more research into the therapeutic properties of alpha-lipoic acid. So far, one small study has shown that supplements of the nutrient help prevent "bad" LDL cholesterol from oxidizing into a form that clogs arteries.

For people with diabetes, alpha-lipoic acid's promise may lie in its ability to relieve diabetic neuropathy, a painful complication that occurs when high blood sugar damages nerve endings. This results in stabbing, tingling, and burning sensations in the feet, legs, and hands, especially at night. "A lot of new evidence suggests that diabetic neuropathy is due in part to oxidative stress, and that people with diabetes have deficient antioxidant capacity," says Aaron Vinik, M.D., Ph.D., director of the Strelitz Diabetes Research Institute at the Eastern Virginia Medical School in Norfolk. Alpha-lipoic acid may replenish that deficiency.

In Europe, preliminary studies of alpha-lipoic acid as a treatment for diabetic neuropathy have been very encouraging, Dr. Vinik says. More information will come from a four-year clinical trial currently underway at several centers in Europe and the United States. In the meantime, a prescription form of alpha-lipoic acid marketed specifically for diabetic neuropathy already is available in Germany.

Other research has shown that alpha-lipoic acid may help regulate blood sugar. A recent well-controlled German study found that 600 milligrams of alpha-lipoic acid a day helped stabilize blood sugar levels in people with type 2 diabetes.

So what's the bottom line? The early evidence supporting the use of alpha-lipoic acid to treat high blood sugar and diabetic neuropathy is quite convincing. Dr. Vinik estimates that as many as 15 percent of endocrinologists in the United States recommend alpha-lipoic acid to their diabetes patients. It appears to cause only mild side effects such as headache and nausea, even at high doses.

As for the other potential health benefits of alpha-lipoic acid, while they make sense biologically, they haven't been confirmed scientifically. That may change in the years ahead.

If you want to try alpha-lipoic acid—with your doctor's approval, of course—your best bet is supplements. You won't get anywhere near a therapeutic dose from foods; seven pounds of spinach, for example, would supply just 1 milligram of alpha-lipoic acid. You need much, much more than that. Experts recommend buying 300-milligram capsules and taking between two and four per day. With a lower-strength supplement, you may end up swallowing as many as twenty-four pills a day to reach the desired dose.

AMERICAN GINSENG: DRUG-FREE BLOOD SUGAR CONTROL

According to some preliminary studies, American ginseng (*Panax quinquefolius*) may help people with type

2 diabetes lower their blood sugar with few side effects. This research was long overdue. Almost all Western-style clinical trials involving herbs took place in Europe—primarily in Germany, where not many people use American ginseng.

Asian ginseng (*Panax ginseng*) can lower blood sugar, too—at least in small animals. In fact, more than four hundred plants appear to improve blood sugar levels. Some are popular remedies in developing countries, where few people can afford conventional diabetes medications. But the effectiveness of these plants remains unproven.

In the case of American ginseng, the first laboratory trials to examine the impact of the herb on blood sugar date back to 1987. Those studies involved mice. More recent research, involving both nondiabetic and type 2 diabetic human subjects, has produced some encouraging results.

Several trials come from Canadian researcher Vladimir Vuksan, Ph.D., and his colleagues at St. Michael's Hospital at the University of Toronto. In one of their studies, people with type 2 diabetes received between three and nine grams of American ginseng at various intervals up to two hours before eating a meal that supplied 25 grams of glucose. Everyone showed notable declines in their postmeal blood sugar levels. What's more, the size of the reduction did not depend on the amount of the herb or the timing of the dosage. In a nutshell, taking at least three grams of American ginseng within two hours of eating lowered postmeal blood sugar by about 20 percent.

Interestingly, a similar study of people without diabetes yielded somewhat different results. This time, the study participants received smaller doses of American ginseng, just one to three grams. Still, they saw drops in their postmeal blood sugar levels. But for them, timing of the dosage was a factor. The herb proved most effective when taken more than forty minutes before a meal; any later, and the herb didn't work nearly as well.

In both studies, the American ginseng did not change premeal, or fasting, blood sugar levels. This is significant, because it means the herb is unlikely to trigger an adverse reaction, in terms of lowering blood sugar too much.

BITTER MELON: NEW HOPE FROM AN ANCIENT REMEDY

Though not widely known in the United States, bitter melon has a long history as a treatment for diabetes in the traditional medicines of China, India, and Africa. It contains several key compounds known as phytonutrients, which appear to act much like sulfonyurea drugs in the body, only without the side effects. Other compounds in bitter melon are close chemical relatives of insulin.

You should be able to find bitter melon, which looks like a shriveled cucumber, in Asian groceries. You may want to try adding it to soup or a stir-fry. Keep in mind, though, that it tastes just like its name suggests. And be careful not to eat the seeds or rind; they're poisonous.

You can buy bitter melon as a juice. But if you

drink too much, you may experience side effects like nausea, vomiting, diarrhea, or hypoglycemia. For this reason, you should use the juice only with the guidance of a naturopathic doctor or licensed herbal practitioner.

CHROMIUM: TROUBLE FROM TOO LITTLE

A trace mineral, chromium can enhance the body's ability to regulate blood sugar, according to Richard A. Anderson, Ph.D., a biochemist for the U.S. Department of Agriculture (USDA) Human Nutrition Research Center in Beltsville, Maryland. Some people with diabetes may benefit from chromium supplements, especially if they test positive for a deficiency. Research has shown that diabetics are more prone to lower blood levels of chromium than nondiabetics.

In one small study, eight people who struggled to control their blood sugar took twenty micrograms of chromium every day. After five weeks, their blood sugar levels fell by as much as 50 percent. On the other hand, readings remained unchanged in those who didn't have blood sugar problems to begin with.

The recommended dosage for people with diabetes is 200 micrograms of chromium a day. People with especially severe blood sugar trouble may need to take more of the mineral, notes Michael Janson, M.D., author of *Dr. Janson's New Vitamin Revolution*.

CINNAMON: A SPICE WITH POTENTIAL

Not long ago, scientists for the USDA Agricultural Research Service decided to test a number of herbs popular in folk medicine to determine whether the plants' active ingredients had any measurable impact on blood sugar. Of more than fifty plant extracts, cinnamon produced the best results in terms of enabling cells to use insulin. Its effects were so promising, in fact, that they prompted a series of clinical trials. This research, which began in 2001, may lead to a patent for a cinnamon extract.

In the meantime, you can use cinnamon straight from your spice rack. Some experts suggest consuming ¼ to 1 teaspoon of ground cinnamon every day. Try stirring it into your oatmeal, orange juice, or coffee.

DANDELION: A DANDY SOLUTION TO OXIDATIVE STRESS

As a common yard weed, dandelion isn't about to win any popularity contests. But as a medicinal herb, it could turn out to be an important contender in the fight against diabetes.

In a Korean study, dandelion successfully reduced blood sugar levels in diabetic dogs. Subsequent research determined that the herb also offsets the free radical damage that may contribute to diabetes complications.

Dandelion appears to offer other benefits as well. Chinese folk healers, for example, use it to treat a host of cancers. Wisely, perhaps, because animal research has shown that dandelion inhibits the conversion of normal cells to cancerous cells in the presence of cancer-causing chemicals. What's more, dandelion appears to stop the growth and formation of tumors. It stimulates cancer-fighting immune cells, too.

Drinking a healthy beverage such as dandelion tea can help increase your well-being one gulp at a time. Brew some every morning by steeping three teaspoons of dried dandelion root in three cups of freshly boiled water for ten minutes, then straining out the herb. Sip the tea throughout the day. Another option: Take two 500-milligram capsules of dried dandelion root three times a day.

GYMNEMA SYLVESTRE: STOPS SUGAR CRAVINGS COLD

Gymnema plays a prominent role in Ayurveda, India's traditional healing discipline. The herb contains a compound, gymnemic acid, that acts directly on the tongue to block the ability to taste sweetness. This may help derail sugar cravings, so you won't be tempted to indulge in treats that could spike your blood sugar. The only caveat is, you must chew the fresh herb or put a drop of the tincture directly on your tongue. Gymnema won't stop cravings if taken in pill or capsule form.

The herb can help control diabetes in another way. Specifically, it appears to stimulate the production of insulin and to enhance the activity of the hormone. Some people have found that once they start taking gymnema, they can reduce their dosage of hypoglycemic medication, if not go off the drug altogether. (Of course, you never should discontinue a prescription or alter a dosage without first consulting your doctor.) For this purpose, experts recommend taking 400 milligrams of gymnema capsules every day.

VITAMIN C: YOU NEED MORE THAN ENOUGH

If you have diabetes, getting extra vitamin C in supplement form is a smart strategy. That's because people with diabetes are prone to high levels of oxidative stress, the kind of cellular damage that can raise your risk for multiple diabetes complications, including heart disease, neuropathy, and blindness. Vitamin C helps repair this damage. As a bonus, it lowers blood sugar by preventing the glucose that's already inside cells from converting to sorbitol, a sugar that can't be used for energy.

The trouble with vitamin C is, if blood sugar rises high enough to be excreted from the body in urine, the vitamin will travel right along with it. But taking extra C in supplement form can help replenish the supply, says Carol Johnston, Ph.D., a vitamin C researcher and professor at Arizona State University East in Mesa. In fact, she believes that vitamin C supplements should be a component of the standard treatment protocol for people with diabetes. She recommends taking 500 to 1,000 milligrams of vitamin C a day, well above the Daily Value, to saturate blood and tissues with the nutrient.

Unfortunately, a sizable segment of the U.S. population—as many as one in three Americans—doesn't get nearly enough vitamin C. "I see it all the time in my research," Dr. Johnston notes. "People who run low on C are more likely to be fatigued and have no

THESE HERBS MAY SAVE YOUR SIGHT

Doctors familiar with herbal medicine sometimes recommend the herbs bilberry and ginkgo to their patients with diabetes. Both herbs improve circulation, which may help lower the risk of retinopathy, a common diabetes complication.

You can find bilberry and ginkgo in health food stores, either freeze-dried or as a tincture. Whichever product you choose, follow the label instructions for proper dosage.

energy for exercise." One possible reason for the shortfall, she says, is that certain foods and beverages may not contain as much vitamin C as we previously thought. As an example, when she tested the vitamin C content of orange juice, she found that the ready-to-drink variety had 70 percent less C than the frozen concentrate.

Because supplements deliver a precise, consistent dose of vitamin C, you can be sure that you're getting enough. Your best bet is to take the suggested 500 to 1,000 milligrams as two or three smaller doses, spread over the course of the day. And don't buy into claims that certain supplements work better than others. Plain old vitamin C, also called ascorbic acid, absorbs just as well as more expensive kinds.

Be aware that the safe upper limit for vitamin C is 2,000 milligrams a day. Taking more than that can cause diarrhea or stomach upset. In fact, in too-large doses, vitamin C can be harmful instead of helpful, cautions Abby Bloch, Ph.D., R.D., past chairperson of the American Cancer Society's committee on nutrition and physical activity.

HELP FROM THE MEDICINE CHEST

If your doctor hasn't suggested it, you may want to ask whether you're a candidate for aspirin therapy. The popular over-the-counter pain reliever has proven to be a potent heart attack preventive, too. It reduces risk by discouraging certain blood cells, called platelets, from sticking together in the arteries.

Amazingly, aspirin therapy appears to work even better for people with diabetes than for those without. That's especially good news for diabetic women, as the incidence of heart attack among this segment of the population has been on the rise in recent years. Your doctor can recommend the right dosage for you.

Anyone with late-stage diabetes should skip vitamin C supplements altogether. They could contribute to kidney failure.

VITAMIN E: INSULIN ENHANCER AND MORE

Like vitamin C, vitamin E is an antioxidant. It not only helps offset the damage caused by oxidative stress, it also supports the proper function of insulin receptor sites on cells.

What's more, vitamin E interferes with a process called glycosylation, in which sugar interacts with protein in a way that alters protein's structure. Experts suspect that glycosylation sets the stage for diabetes complications.

Dr. Janson recommends taking 400 to 800 international units of vitamin E a day. But as with all the other remedies in this chapter, be sure to check with your doctor first—especially if you're on aspirin therapy or using an anti-coagulant medication such as warfarin (Coumadin). The reason: Vitamin E also acts as a blood thinner.

If you have late-stage diabetes, the same caution applies as for vitamin C. Skip the vitamin E supplements, because of the risk of kidney failure.

PART III

Living Well with Diabetes

CHAPTER FIVE

Attitude Matters

Say "diabetes," and the next word that usually comes to mind is "diet," with a capital D. The two seem to go hand-in-hand. Certainly, what you eat—not to mention how often you exercise—can make all the difference in how well you manage your condition.

But according to the latest research, a third factor may influence blood sugar levels just as much. It's emotional health. And at least in terms of diabetes, it hasn't gotten the attention it deserves.

To help bridge this information gap, let's take a closer look at the role of mood and mindset in diabetes self-care. The research to date has made some truly remarkable findings that are destined to change diabetes treatment in the years ahead. By presenting them here, we hope that you can get a head start on lifelong good health.

STRESS: THE BLOOD SUGAR SABOTEUR

While defusing stress makes sense for everyone, it is vital if you have diabetes. Chronic, uncontrolled stress—even the everyday kind brought on by too many responsibilities and not enough time—can mess with your blood sugar and your efforts to keep it in check.

By way of definition, stress occurs when you feel ill-equipped to meet the demands placed on your mind and body. Generally, people associate this perception with negative circumstances, such as illness or problems at the office. But experts say it can just as easily accompany positive situations, like planning a wedding or moving into a new home.

You probably have firsthand experience with the effects of stress: Your neck tenses up, your head hurts, your stomach is in knots, you can't sleep. By recognizing these warning signs early on, you can take steps to address the underlying problem and to shut down your body's stress response.

When you feel tense and anxious, as though you're on an emotional roller coaster, you may not be aware that your blood sugar is taking a ride, too. That's because stress hormones like adrenaline raise your blood sugar to provide a temporary energy boost. It would be a lifesaving reaction if you were, say, being chased by a pack of wild dogs. Then you'd want to be able to run like the wind. The extra blood sugar can help with that.

Thankfully, we don't need to fend off potentially man-eating beasts as our prehistoric ancestors did. Modern stressors tend to be more psychological than physical. So instead of fighting or fleeing, we sit and stew. Our bodies don't use up all the blood sugar that the stress response leaves behind.

Because people who have diabetes don't effectively metabolize blood sugar to begin with, they need to do all they can to minimize the stressors in their lives. The impact of stress on diabetes management is clear. Lois Jovanovic, M.D., an endocrinologist from Santa Barbara, California, who specializes in diabetes in women, reports that her patients typically have the most difficulty controlling their blood sugar during tax week. Other physicians have noticed a pattern of poor results on blood sugar tests among diabetics for up to a month after they experience a death in the family. And diabetes educators caution their clients to carefully monitor their blood sugar levels during illness, since an immune system fighting an infection releases stress hormones that can inhibit insulin's effects.

Stress can undermine diabetes management in another, more indirect way. When you're feeling pressured or overwhelmed, you're more likely to stray from your good eating and exercise habits. That can send your blood sugar spinning out of control. So you have even more reason to be proactive about nipping stressful situations in the bud.

EVERYDAY WAYS TO LIVE STRESS-FREE

Study after study has proven that developing the skills to effectively cope with stress can dramatically improve your ability to keep a lid on blood sugar in trying times. In one particular trial, eighteen people with diabetes lowered their blood sugar levels by 9 to 12 percent through simple relaxation techniques alone.

But these exercises may work best when you're tuned in to your state of mind, says Angele McGrady, Ph.D., lead author of the study and professor at the Medical College of Ohio in Toledo. They didn't appear to help those who were dealing with depression or anxiety in addition to stress.

Then again, some people simply respond better to one relaxation technique over another. Your best bet is to experiment with a variety of exercises to identify those that not only produce the best results but also suit your lifestyle. That way, you'll be more likely to continue using them—ideally, every day.

Just one caveat: Be sure to check in with your doctor before incorporating relaxation techniques into your self-care plan. Your doctor may decide to monitor your blood sugar to see the effects of the exercises you try. If you take medication, you may need to adjust your dosage, so you don't end up with dangerously low blood sugar levels.

With that in mind, feel free to take advantage of the following strategies for maximum relaxation and minimum stress.

Practice deep breathing. Deep breathing is a perfect introductory technique for those new to relaxation, Dr. McGrady says. To try it, begin by sitting in a comfortable chair, leaving your arms and legs uncrossed. Inhale deeply from your abdomen, then exhale, releasing as much air as possible. Relax your muscles as you do. Continue for about fifteen minutes.

Use your ears to unwind. Can't seem to stop your mind from racing? A relaxation tape might help. "Most of us aren't accustomed to sitting quietly, with no thoughts in our heads," Dr. McGrady explains. "We like to have some sound in the background." Recordings from nature, such as ocean waves, not only create a soothing ambience but also pace your breathing. Look for them wherever you buy music tapes or CDs.

Focus on a tranquil scene. In a technique called guided imagery, you use your recall and concentration to conjure a relaxing mental picture. You can achieve virtually the same effect by examining a photo or painting that you find pleasant. "Study it for several minutes, then close your eyes and remember as much as you can," Dr. McGrady says. "Eventually, if you practice enough, you can re-create the image in your mind without first seeing it."

If you spend a lot of time on the computer, you could turn a favorite picture into a screensaver, then use it as a visual cue whenever you need to de-stress. Another option is to listen to a guided imagery tape, in which a soothing voice describes a scene as you close your eyes and imagine it.

Try progressive relaxation. As its name suggests, progressive relaxation involves contracting and relaxing each muscle group in your body. In this way, you learn to consciously control tension, which in turn helps relieve stress. To begin, lie on your back in a comfortable position. Tense and release your fists, then move upward through your arms to your neck and face. Finish with your back and, finally, your legs. Be careful not to squeeze any muscle group so hard that you feel pain, Dr. McGrady cautions.

Take the express route to less stress. For maximum relaxation in minimal time, Dr. McGrady recommends the following "cross-training" technique. First, practice deep breathing for a minute or two. Then proceed to progressive relaxation, tensing and releasing the muscles from your feet up to your head. Continue for ten to fifteen minutes, noticing how each body part feels warm, heavy, and loose after you've worked it.

COPING AS A COUPLE

Anyone who has diabetes will agree that the disease can affect almost every aspect of your life, including your relationship with your spouse. But it needn't come between the two of you. In fact, a recent study from the State University of New York Upstate Medical University shows that a healthy marriage actually can improve your ability to cope with the stress of diabetes.

When researchers interviewed seventy-eight married couples, each with a spouse who used insulin to treat type 1 or type 2 diabetes, they identified distinct differences in the quality of diabetes self-care. Specifically, the diabetics in happy marriages felt comfortable with daily tasks like blood tests and insulin shots. On the other hand, the diabetics in troubled marriages felt emotionally distressed and overwhelmed by their illness.

Experts attribute the differences largely to better communication between the partners in happy marriages. They're more inclined to work together as a team, which can help reduce stress for both of them.

"But in relationships with lots of conflict, people feel alone," explains Paula M. Trief, Ph.D., who co-authored the study with Ruth Weinstock, M.D., Ph.D., of the Joslin Diabetes Center in Syracuse, New York. "The person without diabetes may resent his or her partner's needs. Or the person with diabetes may try to conceal his or her needs."

Of course, you can't control your spouse's feelings about your illness. But you can do your part to sustain the sort of nurturing partnership that makes managing diabetes so much easier. These tips can help.

Encourage your spouse to open up. In marriages where one partner has diabetes, the other may feel overwhelmed by all that goes into treating the disease. Or the person may be worried about the onset of complications down the road. Simply talking through these feelings can help allay fears for both spouses, as well as reinforce the sense of intimacy between them.

Play word association. A spouse who is reluctant to express feelings may enjoy this nonthreatening exercise, which can help initiate a conversation. Each of you writes the word *diabetes* on a piece of paper. Next, spend a few minutes thinking about the word and writing down any phrases or images that come to mind. Then you and your spouse can compare lists and ask questions about each other's notes.

Be clear about your needs. Your spouse may want to help but not know how. Why not offer some suggestions? Perhaps your partner can lend a hand with food shopping or meal preparation, go along for doctor's visits, or just listen. Consider all the options, and talk about what each of you feels most comfortable with.

Use fuzzy math. Long-term relationships seldom are a 50/50 proposition. They're more like 60/60, with both partners doing a little more than their share. So forget about keeping score. It will only eat away at your happiness.

Consider short-term counseling. If diabetes seems to be coming between you and your spouse, you may want to seek guidance from a marriage counselor or a member of the clergy. It may take time, but the two of you can resolve negative feelings that interfere with intimacy.

DEPRESSION: THE BLUES–BLOOD SUGAR CONNECTION

Doctors have known for a long time that depression and diabetes tend to go hand-in-hand. But one question has gone unanswered: Which comes first?

At least one study suggests that in most cases, depression arrives earlier. Researchers looked at dates from the medical records of 1,680 people with newly diagnosed type 2 diabetes and the same number without diabetes. They found that the diabetics had experienced significantly more bouts of depression prior to their diagnoses. In fact, among those with diabetes and depression, the latter condition appeared first three-quarters of the time.

"I'm not sure we can say that depression actually causes diabetes," cautions lead researcher Gregory A. Nichols, Ph.D., senior research associate at Kaiser

WHEN DIABETES DAMPENS DESIRE

Couples living with a major illness such as diabetes often struggle with sexual problems, which can be a significant source of stress. For example, poor blood sugar control can affect a woman's estrogen levels, causing scanty lubrication. Chronically high blood sugar also can lead to recurrent yeast and urinary tract infections—another cause of painful intercourse—and loss of genital sensation, impairing a woman's ability to climax.

Needless to say, such problems can reduce a woman's enthusiasm for sex. Physicians usually recommend lubricants such as Astroglide or Replens to help restore moisture to delicate vaginal tissues.

Diabetes can undermine a man's sexual health, too. In fact, between 50 and 60 percent of men over age 50 who have diabetes experience erectile dysfunction. Generally, damage to nerves and blood vessels is to blame. Either the penis can't respond to arousal signals from the brain or the damaged vessels can't get enough blood into the penis to produce an erection.

A variety of interventions—including the prescription drug Viagra, penile suppositories, penile injections, and vacuum erection devices—can restore erectile function. It definitely is worth a conversation with a doctor, who probably will order a battery of tests to determine the best course of treatment.

Permanente Center for Health Research in Portland, Oregon. He believes both conditions may be linked to a common factor that studies have yet to identify.

For now, if you've been diagnosed with diabetes, Dr. Nichols recommends paying extra attention to your moods. "I'd consider depression a possible warning sign," he says. "If you're feeling depressed, get treated—and get your blood sugar checked, too."

Here's what else you can do.

Put pleasure on your schedule. Every morning, jot down a few enjoyable activities—going for a walk, puttering in the garden, listening to a new CD—that you plan to do during the day. Give these activities the same priority that you would a serious business appointment.

Stay in touch with friends. A British study found that 65 percent of women with depression who met with a volunteer "befriender" for one hour a week experienced a remission of their symptoms, compared with 39 percent of women who didn't get the extra support. That's about the same success rate associated with medication or conventional therapy, notes study author Tirril Harris, Ph.D., a researcher with the Socio-Medical Research Center in London.

Banish negative thoughts. Dwelling on the serious nature of diabetes or the risk of potential complications can deepen a blue mood. But remember, you have a surprising amount of control over the thoughts that flit through your mind. So try turning the negatives into positives. When you tell yourself "I'm in control of my diabetes" or "I show no signs of complications," you diminish your sense of sadness.

Stay in touch with your spirituality. Studies have shown that people who are active in their churches or synagogues and feel a connection to God or some higher power experience fewer bouts of depression.

Know when to seek professional help. If sad feelings intensify or persist, a talk with a counselor could be in order, Dr. McGrady says. Depression—

which is even more common in diabetics than in the general population—is associated with an increased risk of diabetic complications. It also may worsen insulin resistance.

The good news is, people with diabetes usually respond well to treatment for emotional distress. In a study from the Washington University School of Medicine, when type 2 diabetics added cognitive behavioral therapy to their diabetes management, more than 70 percent went into remission from depression. As a bonus, they saw declines in their blood sugar levels. By comparison, those who didn't use therapy experienced increases in their blood sugar levels, and the majority of them continued to suffer from depression.

THE REAL PAYOFF OF EFFECTIVE CONTROL

Hopefully by now, you're convinced that your mood and mindset can have a direct and profound impact on your diabetes self-care. Guess what? The opposite also is true.

According to the results of a new study, maintaining healthy blood sugar levels can enhance your perceived quality of life. For the study, researchers at Harvard University tracked the health status of nearly seven hundred people with type 2 diabetes. After six months on an experimental drug, those with improved blood sugar also reported more energy and vitality, less anxiety, and a better social life. They made fewer doctors' visits, and in general, they felt better about their health. Because the results were so consistent,

COMING TO TERMS WITH A DIABETES DIAGNOSIS

Finding out you have a serious, chronic illness like diabetes can feel overwhelming at first. With these tips, you can minimize your mental stress and improve your chances of a good long-term prognosis.

Allow an adjustment period. After being diagnosed with diabetes, you can expect to experience the same five stages of grieving as a person who has lost a loved one: disbelief/denial, anger, depression/withdrawal, recovery, acceptance. Complicating this process is the anxiety brought on by both high and low blood sugar, as you and your doctor work to identify the best self-care strategies. All told, you may need about a year to adjust to your condition and settle into your management plan. Give yourself this time, knowing you will feel better soon.

Ask questions. Anyone newly diagnosed with diabetes is bound to feel scared and intimidated if they believe that all diabetics go blind or end up on kidney dialysis. But it just isn't true. So try not to get sucked in by hearsay or let your imagination run wild. Instead, express your concerns to your health-care team. They will not only separate myths from reality but also offer invaluable advice for reducing your risk of complications.

Choose a role model. Think of people like 1999 Miss America Nicole Johnson, and blind cyclist and Paralympic gold-medalist Pam Fernandes. Both have type I diabetes, yet they enjoy active, rewarding lifestyles. You can, too!

they support the existence of some physiological connection between healthy blood sugar and overall well-being, notes lead researcher Donald C. Simonson, M.D., associate professor of medicine at Harvard Medical School.

Dr. Simonson and his colleagues believe that any

measures to control blood sugar can have similar feel-good benefits. Here's a trio to start out.

Stick with your program. Even small downward shifts in blood sugar levels can result in enhanced well-being, Dr. Simonson says. So renew your commitment to the diet-and-exercise program prescribed by your doctor. Consider keeping a journal to chart your progress.

Take your medication consistently. After four to eight weeks of drug therapy, most diabetics feel noticeably peppier. Yet a recent study shows that only one-third of people with type 2 diabetes refill their prescriptions often enough to take most of their meds.

Get the latest test. Better control requires better testing. For the most accurate long-term reading of your blood sugar levels, ask your doctor for a glycosylated hemoglobin (HbA1c) test at least every three months, in addition to regular blood sugar screenings.

CHAPTER SIX

The Fitness Factor

If stumbling to the coffeepot at dawn and stretching for the potato chips at night is your idea of staying in shape, you're missing out on a powerful weapon against diabetes: burning calories.

"People with diabetes spend so much time talking about food that they often forget about the other facet of diet, which is expending energy," says David Robbins, M.D., director of research in atherosclerosis and diabetes at Medlantic Research Institute and professor of medicine at George Washington University, both in Washington, D.C. "If you have diabetes, exercise can improve your blood sugar levels." It also makes your body's cells more sensitive to insulin.

Just how important is regular physical activity? Consider the results of one study, in which Swedish researchers assigned forty-one men with type 2 diabetes to a weight-reduction and exercise program. After six years, half of the men no longer experienced diabetes symptoms.

For the same study, one hundred eighty-one men with borderline diabetes followed a similar program to slim down and shape up. After five years, three-quarters of them showed normal blood sugar levels.

According to the American College of Sports Medicine (ACSM), people who are obese and have type 2 diabetes can control their blood sugar better when they work out regularly. What's more, research has shown that increased physical activity can reduce the risk of heart attack, stroke, and other diabetes complications.

The really good news is that any exercise appears to help. Whether you're flying a kite, perfecting your breaststroke, or stacking heavy cans in the pantry, working your muscles requires a lot of energy. This means your muscles must pull glucose from your bloodstream to feed their cells. In fact, for up to two hours after you finish your workout, your liver and muscles are busy clearing glucose out of your blood as they replenish their stores.

For those who are dependent on insulin or diabetes medications, exercise offers a bonus benefit. "At the very least, they will need less medicine," says Robert Hanisch, senior medical exercise physiologist and certified diabetes educator for the Diabetes Treatment Center at Columbia–St. Mary's Hospital in Milwaukee. "And the results are immediate."

Though the effects vary, the average person experiences a 1- to 2-point drop in blood sugar for every minute of physical activity. So ten minutes of aerobic exercise could lower blood sugar by 10 to 20 points—and generally, it will stay at that level until your next meal or snack.

THE BIG BENEFITS OF A LITTLE WEIGHT LOSS

If you have diabetes and you're overweight, shedding those extra pounds ought to be your highest priority. "Increased body mass means a greater demand for insulin to run every cell of the body," explains Denise Faustman, M.D., Ph.D., associate professor of medicine and director of the immunobiology laboratory at Massachusetts General Hospital in Boston. "What's more, since people who are obese generally consume more calories, it further drives up the amount of insulin necessary to process all the extra glucose." This in turn increases the workload of the pancreas, which already is stretched thin trying to rein in out-of-control blood sugar.

Yet, you don't need to lose 50-plus pounds to lower blood sugar to a healthy level. Especially if you have type 2 diabetes, taking off just 5 to 10 percent of your body weight may be enough. And even that range is relative. "I've seen people with type 2 diabetes able to go off insulin after dropping about twenty-five pounds," notes Anne Daly, R.D., C.D.E., a certified diabetes educator and president of health care and education for the American Diabetes Association in Springfield, Illinois.

And slimming down is good for more than your blood sugar. You'll put less stress on your hips and knees when you work out, protecting yourself against osteoarthritis. You'll reduce your risk of heart disease and certain kinds of cancer. You'll have more energy. And you'll just feel better about yourself.

HOW TO STAY SAFE WHILE YOU SWEAT

Of course, if you have diabetes, you should be extra-careful when launching an exercise program, especially if you've been relatively sedentary. Your first step is to schedule an appointment for a complete physical exam—including a stress test if you're over age 35 or you have heart disease as well as diabetes. Then you and your doctor can work together to develop a workout that suits your health status and fitness level. Consider this advice as well.

Test your blood sugar before, during, and after exercise. For diabetics, perhaps the greatest risk of physical activity is having too-high or too-low blood sugar before they begin to exert themselves. That's why regular testing is so important.

If your blood sugar is below 100 mg/dl (milligrams per deciliter), you need to raise it before you begin your workout. Otherwise, it's going to drop even lower. Your best bet is to consume 10 to 15 grams of carbohydrates, such as four ounces of orange juice mixed with four ounces of water, four peanut butter crackers, or half of a banana.

If your blood sugar is above 250 mg/dl, you should check your blood for ketones, metabolic byproducts that occur in abnormally high quantities in uncontrolled diabetes. The presence of ketones means you could need insulin. What's more, you should refrain from exercising, because physical exertion will push your blood sugar even higher. No ketones? You probably can work out, provided you lower your blood sugar first. In most cases, several units of short-acting insulin will do the trick. Ask your doctor what's best for you.

Once you start exercising, the harder you push yourself, the more glucose your muscle cells will pull from your bloodstream. For this reason, you ought to check your blood sugar about every twenty minutes—especially if you're a beginning exerciser, you're working with extra intensity, or you're practicing tight control. Check after you finish your workout, too. Because you will have used up so much glucose, you may be able to reduce your dosage of insulin, says Lois Jovanovic, M.D., an endocrinologist who specializes in diabetes in women. Your diabetes educator or another health care practitioner can explain how to adjust your insulin based on your blood-sugar tests.

Be ready with a blood-sugar booster, just in case. What you choose really depends on how hard you'll be working out. Effective pick-me-ups range from a handful of raisins or jelly beans to commercial glucose tablets, sold over-the-counter in pharmacies. Be sure to stash them in a secure place on your body, so you have them when you need them.

Let your activity determine where you inject insulin. Since your muscles are more efficient at using insulin when you're exercising, you should avoid injecting the hormone near a muscle that you're working especially hard. The muscle could take up insulin *too* efficiently, setting the stage for hypoglycemia, says Anne Daly, R.D., C.D.E., a certified diabetes educator and president of health care and education for the American Diabetes Association in Springfield, Illinois. For example, if you're planning a bike ride, you're better off taking the injection in your abdomen rather than your thigh. But if you're gearing up for a tennis match, use your thigh rather than your arm.

Keep an eye on your feet. People who have diabetes often lose sensation in their feet. And because the disease slows the healing process, any blisters or other sores are more prone to infection. This is why even recreational athletes who are diabetic must take extra precautions, Daly says.

If you have diabetes, you should inspect your feet on a daily basis, whether or not you work out. Look for signs of developing blisters, corns, and calluses. They may require special care, including treatment by a podiatrist.

To prevent problems in the first place, keep your feet clean and dry, especially between your toes. Always wear good-quality socks, with the seams where they should be, and good-fitting shoes. Shake out your shoes before putting them on, since even a small pebble could do damage.

What if you hurt one of your feet despite your best efforts to protect them? Try switching to a non-weight-bearing activity, such as swimming or using a rowing machine, for the duration of the healing process. Depending on the severity of the sore, you may be able to ride a stationary bike or walk for short periods of time. Check with your doctor or podiatrist, Daly advises.

Account for any complications. For example, if you have diabetic retinopathy—an eye disease that can lead to vision loss—you should avoid exercise positions in which your heart is higher than your head. And steer clear of heavy lifting, which can elevate pressure in your eyes.

No matter what complications you may be dealing with, your doctor or a physical therapist can recommend a physical activity you can do safely. "I know an endocrinologist who has stroke patients and leg amputees meet in his office to practice 'conducting the orchestra' or 'directing the choir,' " says Frank Schwartz, M.D., clinical associate professor of medicine, endocrinology, and metabolism at West Virginia University School of Medicine in Parkersburg. "After twenty minutes, they're exhausted, and they get a real aerobic workout."

READY, SET . . . SHAPE UP!

Contrary to conventional wisdom, you don't need to punish your body to reap the benefits of physical activity. Sure, you want to challenge yourself. But you don't want to go overboard. That's true even if you don't have diabetes—and especially if you do.

The fact is, regular, moderate exercise yields just as good results as an all-out effort. So once you have your doctor's okay, follow these tips to make working out a habit.

First and foremost, use common sense. For safety's sake, find someone to work out with you. In the absence of willing recruits, consider joining a fitness facility that's equipped to handle medical emergencies. And by all means, wear a medical ID tag. It alerts medical personnel, among others, that you have diabetes. So if you can't speak for yourself in the event of an emergency, you're sure to get proper care.

Ease into it. Not accustomed to exercise? Don't sweat it. Begin with a low-impact, low-intensity activity such as walking. And go at a comfortable pace, Hanisch advises. If you push yourself too hard, you won't enjoy it and you'll be less likely to stick with it. "Your blood sugar can drop even when you're walking very slowly," he notes. (We'll talk more about starting a walking program a bit later in the chapter.)

Strive for five. According to ACSM guidelines, everyone with diabetes should work out for ten to fifteen minutes at least three nonconsecutive days each week. Hanisch suggests gradually building up to thirty minutes of physical activity most days of the week. "Consistency is key," he notes. Whether you hike, bike, jog, or swim, working out five days a week will produce optimum results, including long-term physical changes. After two to three months of consistent physical activity, you likely will be more sensitive to insulin, which means you'll need less medicine, he says.

Join the 1,000 club. The ACSM recommends that people with type 2 diabetes burn at least 1,000 calories a week through daily physical activity. Let's say you weigh about 150 pounds. You'd burn about 166 calories by walking briskly for thirty minutes. Do it five days a week, and you'll be close to the 1,000-calorie mark. The rest of your daily activities will more than make up the difference.

Invest in a pedometer. If you want to get a clearer picture of just how active you are, use a pedometer to track how many steps you take. Research has shown that people who incorporate a thirty-minute workout into their daily routines accumulate about 10,000 steps, while those who work in offices average between 2,000 and 4,000 steps. A pedometer can be a very effective motivational tool, because you're self-monitoring. According to fitness experts, people who self-monitor are more likely to reach their exercise goals than people who do not.

Lift with care. Strength training can help build muscle. But people with long-standing diabetes, and especially those with diabetes-related eye disease, should use very light weights—in the range of one to five pounds—and do lots of repetitions. Heavy weights could injure weakened eye muscles, Hanisch notes. You'll know you've chosen the right weight if you can perform an exercise with proper technique and minimal effort. If in doubt, choose a lighter weight.

Be a morning person. Working out in the A.M. can hold down blood sugar all day long. You'll still experience fluctuations in your blood sugar levels after meals. But by starting your day with a thirty-minute walk, you can keep your blood sugar 30 points lower than it might otherwise be, Hanisch says.

That's not the only reason to plan your exercise sessions for first thing in the morning. Fitness experts note that at that time of day, family responsibilities and job demands are less likely to derail your workouts.

Make an appointment to be active. Another favorite strategy of fitness experts is to schedule time for exercise—even blocking out your workouts in your calendar, if you need to. Then you're more likely to follow through on your good intentions.

Drink up, even if you're not thirsty. Dehydration can affect blood sugar levels, so staying well-hydrated during exercise is especially important for people with diabetes. Drink sixteen ounces (two glasses) of water two hours before exercising, then keep sipping during your workout. Unless you're exercising for more than an hour, stick with water instead of juices, sports drinks, and other fluids high in concentrated carbohydrates.

Monitor your intensity. If you feel like you're pushing too hard, you probably are. Ease up, or stop altogether if you feel dizzy or faint. That's your cue to check your blood sugar. Drink plenty of water, too.

Pay particular attention to central fat. If you had to tailor your workout to just one area of body fat, you'd be smart to pick your belly, Dr. Schwartz says. The reason: Insulin resistance is associated with and contributes to abdominal obesity. Several studies have shown that losing fat deep in the abdominal region can lower blood sugar better than losing fat anywhere else.

Of course, working any muscle will improve insulin's efficiency, and losing any fat will reduce the risk of diabetes complications. Aerobic exercise can help on both counts. It's best for reducing abdominal fat.

BEATING DIABETES, ONE STEP AT A TIME

All kinds of activities can provide a good aerobic workout. But none is as easy or as safe as walking. After all, you're just putting one foot in front of the other. You don't need to invest in fancy equipment or a health club membership. You don't even need to wait for good weather. Indoors, you can stride on a treadmill or take laps around the nearest mall. Outside, the sky is the limit.

Best of all, while walking delivers all the benefits of aerobic exercise, it's gentle on your knees, hips,

IN SEARCH OF THE PERFECT SHOE

While walking requires minimal equipment, the one essential—especially for people with diabetes—is proper footwear. Experts recommend shopping for shoes with three criteria in mind: flexibility, toebox, and weight.

An appropriately flexible shoe should bend where your foot naturally bends: at the ball, not in the middle. For maximum comfort during your workouts, you should have enough room in the toebox to properly push off with each step—ideally, a thumb's width between your longest toe and the tip of the shoe. Consider the overall weight, too. Styles with extremely thick cushioned soles aren't necessarily good for walking.

Of course, if you have been diagnosed with diabetic neuropathy, talk with your podiatrist before you buy. He can recommend brands and styles for your particular needs.

and back. So you're less likely to experience the sort of injury that could derail even the most well-intentioned exercise program.

Toward a Sleeker Physique

What if you want to slim down? Well, walking a mile at a moderate pace burns about 100 calories. Since 3,500 calories equals a pound, you could take off a full pound of fat in a little more than a month. The farther and faster you walk, the more you'll lose.

That said, be careful not to do too much too soon, especially if you've been relatively inactive or you need to drop at least 50 pounds. Start out by walking for twenty minutes a day, fast enough that your breathing becomes just a bit labored. You should be able to carry on a conversation without gasping for air.

Try to go the entire twenty minutes without stopping. If it's too much, slow down and rest after ten minutes, then continue on. After a few workouts, you probably will find that you feel great at the end of twenty minutes—like you could walk even more. But don't, at least not for the first three weeks. Stick with the twenty minutes per session.

Walk This Way

To maximize the health-enhancing benefits of your walking program, follow these tips from Kate Larsen, a walking instructor and certified group fitness instructor in Minneapolis.

Learn the heel-to-toe roll. Think of your big toe as a Go button for moving forward and gaining momentum with every step. To press Go, you need to push off from your heel, roll along the outside of your foot, and then push through your big toe. The rest of your toes remain relaxed. This technique takes practice, but it can make a big difference in the efficiency of your stride.

Squeeze your glutes. Contract your glute (buttock) muscles and lift them up and back, as though you were pinching a $50 bill between them. This helps strengthen and tone your glutes. Try to maintain this deep muscle contraction while you walk. It might be difficult at first, but it gets easier over time.

"Zip up" your abs. With every step, imagine that you're zipping up a tight pair of jeans. Stand tall and pull your abdominal muscles up and in. You can do this even when you're not walking. It strengthens your abs and your lower back muscles, too.

Pump your arms. For proper arm movement, stand tall and drop your shoulders, squeezing your shoulder blades behind you. Then slide your elbows back and forth with each step, as though you're holding a pair of ski poles in your hands. The movement should be smooth and strong, with your arms passing the outside of your hips.

Perfect your posture. Think how you'd react if someone poured ice down your back. You'd lift your chest and push back your shoulders. That's how you should carry yourself when practicing good posture.

Hold your head up. As you walk, set your gaze about ten feet ahead of you. Try wearing a baseball cap with the visor level to the horizon. Then you have to look up just enough to see where you're going. It keeps your neck in proper alignment.

Keep your mind in the moment. Try not to replay the events of the day while you're walking. Instead, maintain a state of relaxed awareness by paying attention to how you're breathing and how your body feels. Tell yourself that you're getting healthier, stronger, and leaner with every step.

Above all, enjoy your workouts. All this may seem like a lot to remember. But it will become second nature with time and practice. In the meantime, find ways to spice up your walking program. Choose several different routes and switch among them. Buy a new exercise outfit. Slip on a headset and listen to your favorite music, but only when you're indoors. Otherwise, you might tune out important sounds, like traffic noises.

CHAPTER SEVEN

Nutrition Basics

The link between diet and diabetes has been known for centuries. Unfortunately, the nutritional advice wasn't always the best. As early as 1500 B.C., Middle Easterners pondered whether consuming fruit, wheat, and sweet beer would dry up the excessive urination caused by diabetes. In the eighteenth century A.D., physicians advocated a protein-only plan. As recently as 1900, near-starvation was the treatment of choice.

These days, nobody recommends beer, copious amounts of protein, or an empty plate to control diabetes. Nevertheless, proper nutrition is an important component of any diabetes self-care plan. How important? Consider this statistic: As many as two-thirds of people with type 2 (non-insulin-dependent) diabetes can manage the disease through diet and exercise alone, according to James Anderson, M.D., professor of medicine and clinical nutrition in the Division of Endocrinology and Metabolism at the University of Kentucky College of Medicine in Lexington.

Even for diabetics who depend on medication, diet

can make a world of difference. In a study at the University of California, Los Angeles, six hundred fifty-two people with type 2 diabetes followed a low-fat, high-carbohydrate eating plan for three weeks. Most of the participants also started a walking program. At the end of the three weeks, 71 percent of those taking oral drugs and 39 percent of those using insulin injections no longer needed their medicine.

Perhaps the best news of all for anyone with diabetes is that the so-called diabetic diet isn't what it used to be. Eating to control blood sugar is much more individualized and much less restrictive than in the past. "There's no need for special diabetic food. There's no one-size-fits-all eating plan," says Anne Daly, R.D., C.D.E., a certified diabetes educator and president of health care and education for the American Diabetes Association in Springfield, Illinois. "Just because a person with diabetes eats the same thing for lunch every day doesn't mean you'll have to follow such a monotonous diet."

EATING YOUR WAY

The fact is, everyone with diabetes experiences the disease in a unique way. Each person has a specific set of risk factors, symptoms, and complications—not to mention a distinct mindset and lifestyle. All these variables influence the ability to effectively manage diabetes, and so help determine the structure and components of an ideal eating plan.

Consider that while eight in ten people with diabetes are overweight, two in ten are not. Four in ten may have high levels of LDL (low-density lipoprotein) cholesterol, the "bad" kind that raises the risk of heart disease and stroke. But six in ten may not. For one person, restricting sugary treats might be as easy as a shrug and a "no thanks" when the dessert tray passes by. Another may feel that life without sweets just isn't worth living.

This is why experts have developed a number of eating plans specifically for diabetes. Each plan is scientifically proven to help control blood sugar. You and your doctor should choose the one that best matches your diabetes "profile." Then you can tweak the plan as necessary to accommodate your unique needs—whether you have high cholesterol, for example, or you want to lose a few pounds.

Some people do best with a highly structured, day-by-day eating plan. But for others, "just one or two small changes might be all that's necessary to have big success in controlling diabetes," says Susan Thom, R.D., a nutritionist and certified diabetes educator who owns Nutri-flex, a Cleveland-based consulting company.

Indeed, even small changes can help rein in blood sugar and lower the risk of heart disease and other diabetes-related complications. "One woman who came to me was drinking six cans of sugary cola a day," Thom says. "She decided to switch to diet soft drinks, which cut almost 1,000 calories a day. She lost weight, and her blood sugar dropped to normal in two weeks."

THE RIGHT FOODS AT THE RIGHT TIMES

While diabetes diets take many forms, most adhere to a few core principles. Among them: When and how much you eat is just as important as what you eat. By consuming about the same amount of food at about the same time every day, you keep your blood sugar from fluctuating wildly, explains Ann Zerr, M.D., clinical director of the National Center of Excellence in Women's Health at Indiana University School of Medicine in Indianapolis.

Both bunching your mealtimes and skipping meals can cause fluctuations in blood sugar that are tough on your body. Instead, try to allow four to five hours between breakfast and lunch and five to six hours between lunch and dinner, with a healthy snack at regular intervals between meals. It can make a big difference in your blood sugar levels.

As far as what you eat, experts generally recommend maintaining an ideal balance of carbohydrates, proteins, and fats at every meal. Of course, what's "ideal" can vary from one person to the next. The 7-day menu plan in Chapter 8, designed for weight loss and blood sugar control, slashes the average carbohydrate intake by at least half—from 248-plus grams to 125. You may be able to exceed that limit without affecting your blood sugar.

On the other hand, you should keep a lid on fat—especially saturated fat, which can further raise your risk of heart disease. "In general, high-fat diets increase insulin resistance," Dr. Anderson explains.

"They also contribute to overweight and obesity."

You can get a jump on trimming the fat from your diet just by eating more fish and skinless chicken and less red meat. When you're hungry for red meat, choose a leaner cut and stick with a six-ounce serving. You also might try the following ingredient substitutions in your cooking:

- Sauté with water or low-salt broth instead of oil or butter. Use enough liquid to keep food from sticking to the pan, adding more as necessary.
- Swap low-fat or skim milk for whole milk.
- In recipes that don't require cooking, replace sour cream with equal parts low-fat yogurt and low-fat cottage cheese, beaten until smooth.
- Trade one whole egg for two egg whites plus a tablespoon of vegetable oil. Or use an egg substitute.

Your doctor or a nutritionist can help decide on the best mix of carbs, proteins, and fats to effectively manage your diabetes. For your part, you may want to keep a written record of your food intake and your blood sugar levels, so you can see whether a particular food affects your blood sugar for better or for worse. This can be helpful whether you're starting a new eating plan, adjusting your mealtimes, or even launching a new exercise program (remember, physical activity lowers blood sugar).

FIBER'S ROLE IN BLOOD SUGAR CONTROL

Along with balancing carbs, proteins, and fats, people with diabetes need to get plenty of fiber—between 20

CALORIES COUNT, TOO

When discussing your eating plan with your doctor or nutritionist, be sure to ask about your optimum calorie intake. You should be getting enough to maintain a healthy weight. If you're heavier than you should be, you can either trim calories from your diet or burn more calories through exercise. Ideally, you'll do a combination of the two. For every 3,500 calories you eliminate, you'll lose one pound.

Keep in mind that your body's energy demands, and therefore its calorie needs, will change over time. Still, what seems to trip up most people is not needing fewer calories than they thought but taking in more calories than they realize. "Some people try to live on soups and salads, believing they're on a low-calorie diet when in fact they're eating high-calorie cream soups and salads with dressing," says Anne Daly, R.D., C.D.E., a certified diabetes educator and president of health care and education for the American Diabetes Association in Springfield, Illinois. "Every calorie counts, including those in garnishes and condiments."

and 35 grams a day, Daly says. That's roughly 10 to 20 grams more than the average American consumes.

The beauty of fiber is that it helps "neutralize" the effects of carbohydrates on blood sugar. In fact, if you eat a food that contains at least 5 grams of fiber per serving, you can deduct that amount from the total carbohydrates because it won't contribute to the formation of glucose, Daly says.

In a study at the University of Texas Southwestern Medical Center, people who increased their fiber intakes to 50 grams per day lowered their blood sugar by 10 percent in just 6 weeks. This reduction is comparable to some diabetes medications. To get 50 grams of fiber, just aim for a total of thirteen servings of fruits, vegetables, beans, and grains per day. Among the best sources, per one-cup serving:

Granola	12.8 grams
Chickpeas	12.5 grams
Oat bran	11.4 grams
Oatmeal	9.6 grams
Lima beans	9.0 grams
Raisins	6.6 grams
Kiwi	6.0 grams
Corn	4.6 grams
Oranges	4.3 grams
Blueberries	3.9 grams

Oat bran, beans, and fresh fruits such as apples and pears are especially rich in soluble fiber, the kind that has the greatest impact on both blood sugar and cholesterol. "But Mother Nature provides at least a modest amount of soluble fiber in most foods," Dr. Anderson notes. "So you'll be getting some no matter what you eat."

Increasing your fiber intake does have a couple of caveats. First, you must do it gradually, so your colon can adjust. Otherwise, you may experience cramping and gas, among other mild but uncomfortable digestive complaints, says Belinda M. Smith, R.D., research dietitian for the Metabolic Research Group at the Veterans Affairs Medical Center in Lexington, Kentucky.

To ease the transition to a high-fiber diet, Smith recommends eating a high-fiber cereal for breakfast three or four days one week. The next week, add a little more fiber—by eating fresh fruit instead of drinking juice, for example. The third week, go up another notch, perhaps by substituting beans for ground beef in a recipe or by eating an extra serving of vegetables with a meal.

Don't feel obligated to stick with this timetable. The best approach, Smith says, is to adjust to one change before moving on to another. "I've seen people go hog-wild on oat bran muffins, only to end up with real discomfort," she notes. "Slower definitely is better."

The second caveat for increasing your fiber intake is to drink copious amounts of water—at least eight eight-ounce glasses each day. This is because fiber absorbs tremendous amounts of fluid. It couldn't do its job otherwise.

Can't swallow that much water? Sugar-free beverages like coffee, tea, and diet sodas count toward the recommended fluid intake. But fruit juices and sugary drinks don't. "They're carbohydrates, which means they can raise your blood sugar," Thom says.

DRINK TO YOUR HEALTH WITH CARE

While we're on the subject of beverages, you may be wondering, What about alcohol? Most experts agree that in general, moderate alcohol consumption—no more than one or two drinks a day—won't cause any harm. But if you have diabetes, you must exercise caution.

You see, because alcohol is a toxin, your liver wants to clear it from your blood as quickly as pos-

SODIUM SENSE AND SUBSTITUTIONS

Even though sodium doesn't play a role in diabetes, you may need to watch your intake if you have high blood pressure. Otherwise, it could aggravate an already increased risk for heart disease.

Experts recommend limiting daily sodium consumption to no more than 2,400 milligrams. Those with kidney disease should aim even lower—no more than 2,000 milligrams.

Perhaps the best strategy for reducing your sodium intake is to cut back on salty foods like pickles, cheese, bacon, canned soups, and salad dressings. And instead of seasoning your meals with salt, reach for spices like turmeric and fennel. They add flavor, and they lower blood sugar to boot.

In fact, a number of spices appear to make fat cells more responsive to insulin. At the top of the list is cinnamon, which in studies has produced a twentyfold increase in glucose metabolism.

sible. This can be a problem in combination with diabetes, because alcohol essentially distracts the liver from its glucose-regulating functions.

Normally, when your blood sugar begins to drop, your liver intervenes, dispatching glucose into the bloodstream. But it won't do that until it gets rid of all the alcohol. In the meantime, your blood sugar could dip too low—especially if you haven't eaten, you're exercising, or you're taking insulin or oral diabetes medications. The danger is, you may think you're feeling a buzz from the alcohol when in fact you're slipping into hypoglycemia.

When you want to have a drink, your best bet is to pair it with a meal or snack to counteract the effects on blood sugar. And limit yourself to one—preferably a light beer, a dry wine, or a mix of alcohol and diet soda.

A NEW VIEW OF SUGAR

When first diagnosed with diabetes, most people automatically assume that they can never eat sweets again. True, sugar has a long-standing reputation as white poison, at least in the diabetes community. But in recent years, the American Diabetes Association has taken the bold step of relaxing the "no-sugar" clause in its nutrition guidelines. The organization made its decision based on twelve studies, all of which showed that the majority of people do not experience the dangerous spike in glucose once attributed to eating sweets.

"People with blood sugar trouble still need to be mindful of the sugar and other carbohydrates in their diets," Daly says. "But if someone wants to end a meal with dessert, we can explain how to do it safely." A type 1 diabetic might test her reaction to the sweet and then adjust her insulin dose, while a type 2 diabetic could subtract a few points from her daily "carbohydrate exchange" quota. For those with hypoglycemia, combining a sugary food with protein or fat can help slow digestion.

Still, experts say, you ought to consider whether indulging in sweets really is worth the dietary tradeoff. Even though a small piece of cake may be the carbohydrate equivalent of a slice of whole-wheat bread topped with a teaspoon of margarine, it isn't nearly as filling. What's more, it could be much

CORNSTARCH, ANYONE?

Cornstarch may be the perfect food for people with diabetes. It provides enough sugar to prevent hypoglycemia, but it's digested exceptionally slowly, which helps protect against hyperglycemia. The catch is, it works only when it's eaten in raw form.

You can get raw cornstarch from diabetic foods like Extend Bar, Gluc-O-Bar, and NiteBite—all sold over the counter in pharmacies. According to some experts, these bars make a good nighttime snack for those who want to keep their blood sugar from plummeting in the middle of the night.

higher in fat. "You need to weigh the pluses and minuses," agrees Davida Kruger, R.N., senior vice-president of the ADA. "If I had pie and cake every day, I'd be obese. And I wouldn't get the key nutrients found in fruits, vegetables, and other carbohydrates."

If you're watching your sugar consumption, be aware that the sweet stuff takes many forms—and that all of them count toward your daily sugar quota. Read ingredients lists for sorbitol, xylitol, mannitol, and anything ending in-*ose*, such as dextrose, fructose (also called levulose), maltose, and lactose. These are chemical variations of sugar. Similarly, molasses, corn syrup, confectioners' sugar, cane juice, and maple syrup are considered sucrose. Be sure to account for them when you tally the total carbohydrates in a meal or snack.

If artificial sweeteners don't upset your stomach, you can use saccharine, aspartame, acesulfame potassium, or sucralose instead of sugar. These substitutes don't add calories or raise blood sugar.

PART IV

Eat to Beat Diabetes

CHAPTER EIGHT

Seven Days to Better Blood Sugar Control

If you're overweight and you've been diagnosed with diabetes, your doctor may have recommended unloading those extra pounds. And for good reason: Slimming down by just ten pounds can help improve insulin function and rein in wayward blood sugar levels. It even can reduce dependence on insulin or oral diabetes medications.

But what sort of eating plan can help melt away fat and manage diabetes? Since your carbohydrate intake directly influences your blood sugar levels, a low-carb plan could be the answer.

The principles of low-carb eating are simple: Minimize sweets and refined grains; eat more proteins and high-fiber foods; and stick with sensible portions. For many people, this approach helps normalize blood sugar and curbs the impulse to overeat. As a bonus, it reduces the risk of heart disease and certain cancers.

Still, low-carb eating isn't for everyone. Be sure to talk with your doctor or a nutritionist before trying the plan in this chapter.

WHAT IS A SERVING?

Thanks to the gargantuan platefuls of food that many restaurants serve these days, we Americans have become accustomed to eating more than we should. The average take-out bagel is at least twice the size it ought to be. Even the typical supermarket potato is larger than what experts recommend.

To succeed on a low-carbohydrate eating plan—or any eating plan, for that matter—you need to pay attention to your serving sizes. Use this list for reference.

STARCHES
- 1 slice whole wheat bread
- ½ whole wheat bagel or muffin
- ½ cup cooked whole grain cereal, pasta, brown rice, or other whole grain
- ½ cup cooked beans, corn, potatoes, rice, or sweet potatoes

VEGETABLES
- ½ cup raw, chopped, or cooked vegetables
- ¾ cup vegetable juice
- 1 cup raw leafy greens

FRUITS
- 1 small to medium piece of fruit
- 1 cup whole strawberries or melon cubes
- ½ cup canned or cut fruit
- ¾ cup fruit juice
- ¼ cup dried fruit

PROTEINS
- 1 ounce cooked lean beef, pork, lamb, skinless poultry, fish, or shellfish
- 1 egg

DAIRY
- 1 cup fat-free milk
- 1 cup fat-free or low-fat unsweetened yogurt
- 1 ounce hard cheese (preferably reduced-fat)
- ½ cup low-fat ricotta cheese or cottage cheese
- ¾ cup unsweetened soy milk

NUTS
- 1 ounce nuts without shell
- 2 tablespoons unsweetened peanut butter

UNSATURATED FATS
- 1 teaspoon oil (such as olive, canola, walnut, or flaxseed oil)
- 1 teaspoon regular mayonnaise
- 1 tablespoon low-fat mayonnaise
- 1 tablespoon oil-and-vinegar dressing
- 5 large olives
- ⅛ medium avocado

SATURATED FATS
- 1 teaspoon butter
- 1 slice bacon
- 1 ounce salt pork
- 1 tablespoon heavy cream
- 1 tablespoon cream cheese
- 2 tablespoons sour cream
- 2 tablespoons shredded unsweetened coconut

THE LOW-CARB BREAKTHROUGH

While the low-carb movement has received a lot of attention in recent years, it actually got its start in Paleolithic times. The diet of our caveman ancestors consisted primarily of meats, vegetables, fruits, nuts, and berries. Modern staples like sweets and snack foods didn't exist back then.

The medical community didn't pay much attention to the health effects of carbohydrate restriction until the 1920s, when doctors began recommending low-carb diets as a treatment for intractable epilepsy. Fast-forward another thirty to forty years, and the American public was getting its first taste of the low-carb phenomenon. In the 1960s, Dr. Irwin Stillman touted his low-carb eating plan in a widely read book and on late-night television. A decade later, Dr. Robert Atkins would defy conventional nutritional wisdom and generate intense controversy with his low-carb "diet revolution."

The 1980s and 1990s produced several variations on the low-carb theme, including the Scarsdale Diet, the Zone, Sugar Busters, Protein Power, and the Carbohydrate Addict's Diet. All of these eating plans deliver on their promise to take off extra pounds. But some require complete elimination of certain foods, including healthy ones. As a result, they may be nutritionally inadequate, if not nearly impossible to sustain for a lifetime.

With the eating plan presented here, you won't need to empty your refrigerator and cupboards of all things carbohydrate. In fact, you're more than welcome to continue enjoying carbs like pastas, grains, and even potatoes. Nothing is completely off-limits. And you can adopt the plan at your own pace, based on your motivation to change your eating habits.

In developing the plan, we've drawn on some key principles shared by virtually all low-carb diets.

We've also incorporated the latest research that helps explain why the low-carb approach is so effective for weight loss and blood sugar control. But we know you want more than a plan that works. You want a plan that satisfies your appetite and leaves room for the foods you love. This is it!

NOT ALL CARBS ARE EQUAL

Realistically, you couldn't possibly eliminate all carbohydrates from your diet. Nor would you want to. The fact is, you couldn't survive without them.

Like proteins and fats, carbohydrates are a macronutrient necessary to sustain life. But eating too many carbs can cause weight gain and adversely affect your health. Of course, eating too much of any food can raise the risk of certain health problems. But the story surrounding carbohydrates is a bit more complicated than that.

Carbohydrates encompass a broad range of sugars, starches, and fibers. For the most part, they fall into one of two categories: refined and unrefined. Of the two, refined carbs are much less healthy. In fact, numerous studies have identified a diet high in refined carbohydrates as a risk factor for diabetes as well as heart disease and certain cancers. Among the most common items in this category:

- Any ingredient ending in *-ol*, such as sorbitol
- Any ingredient ending in *-ose*, such as dextrose
- Maple syrup
- Soft drinks

- Sweetened yogurt
- Table sugar

In contrast, unrefined carbohydrates may help reduce the risk of heart disease and cancer, among other health problems. They also play a role in regulating blood sugar. All of the following qualify as unrefined carbs:

- Amaranth
- Arrowroot
- Beans
- Buckwheat
- Fruits
- Fruit juices
- Milk
- Peas
- Plain yogurt
- Potatoes
- Quinoa
- Sweet potatoes
- Tapioca
- Vegetables
- Whole grains (including wheat, oats, barley, and rye)
- Whole grain breads, cereals, and pastas

As you might have guessed from these two lists, unrefined carbs have much greater nutritional value than their refined counterparts. In particular, they're packed with fiber, both soluble and insoluble. In Chapter 7, we discussed how fiber—especially the soluble kind—can help lower blood sugar and cholesterol. It also supports weight loss by slowing the rate of carbohydrate absorption. Remember, too, that because fiber creates a feeling of fullness, you're less inclined to overeat.

UNDERSTANDING THE GLYCEMIC INDEX

So just how do carbohydrates affect your blood sugar, not to mention your waistline? Once in your body, all carbs—from the sucrose in table sugar to the starch in a bagel—convert to glucose, the primary source of cellular energy. By comparison, only 58 percent of proteins and 10 percent of fats turn into glucose. And with carbs, the process takes just a fraction of the time. This is why carbohydrates have a reputation as energy foods. It's also why people with diabetes drink orange juice or take glucose tablets when their blood sugar starts to dip.

But while all carbohydrates convert to glucose and ultimately raise blood sugar, they do it at varying rates. Now, you might think that refined carbs change to glucose quickly, while unrefined carbs go more slowly. Surprisingly, this isn't always the case.

In the early 1980s, researchers developed a numeric system to quantify the effects of carbohydrate-containing foods on blood sugar levels. Called the glycemic index (GI), it ranks carbs by how quickly they raise blood sugar within two to three hours of a meal. The numbers range from 1 to 100, with 100 reserved for pure glucose. The higher the number assigned to a food, the faster that food breaks down and raises blood sugar. Anything with a rating of 55 or

LABEL READING FOR THE CARB-SAVVY

With the advent of the "Nutrition Facts" label, consumers finally could evaluate and compare the nutritional profiles of various foods. Still, the information on carbohydrate content can be confusing. Use these tips to interpret the label lingo.

1. **Check the serving size.** This number appears right at the top of the label, because it's the basis for all the rest of the nutritional data. If you eat more than the stated serving size, you need to increase the rest of the figures proportionately.
2. **Read the "As Prepared" column.** Some packaged foods require the addition of other ingredients, like milk or eggs. You can find out whether this alters the carbohydrate content of a food by assessing the "As Prepared" figures.
3. **Stay to the left.** Look at the total calories, grams, and milligrams that appear on the left side of the label. The "% Daily Value" on the right side is based on 2,000 calories a day, which may not be what you're eating.
4. **Pay extra attention to "Total Carbohydrate."** This is the most important figure when you're watching your carb intake. It represents the sum of the sugars, starch, soluble fiber, and insoluble fiber in a particular food. Some labels also will have separate listings for sugar and fiber. In general, you should stick with foods that will balance your overall carbohydrate intake for the day or week.
5. **Convert grams of sugar to teaspoons.** Most people are better able to visualize teaspoons than grams. It's a simple calculation: Just divide the number of grams listed on the label by 4. Most experts recommend consuming no more than ten teaspoons of sugar per day.
6. **Strive for fiber.** Fiber helps slow the absorption of glucose from carbohydrate-containing foods. Aim for 20 to 35 grams per day, especially if you have diabetes.
7. **Go pro(tein).** Depending on your calorie intake and weight-loss goals, you should be getting between 75 and 150 grams of protein per day. Keep that in mind when choosing foods.

below is said to be low GI, because it causes only a little blip in blood sugar levels. Foods considered high GI, 56 or above, send blood sugar soaring.

All of the following fall into the low GI category:

- Breads: Pumpernickel, sourdough
- Grains: Barley, parboiled rice, bulgur, kasha
- Pastas: Angel hair, linguine, and other thin strands; bean threads (cellophane noodles); whole grain spaghetti
- Cereals: Rice bran, unsweetened high-fiber (all bran) cereals
- Vegetables: All except those listed as high GI
- Fruits: Cherries, grapes, apples, peaches, pears, plums, strawberries, oranges, dried apricots
- Protein foods: Unsweetened peanut butter, beans, eggs, unsweetened soy milk
- Snacks: Cheese, nuts, olives
- Miscellaneous: Low-fat yogurt; foods sweetened with sucralose, fructose, saccharine, or aspartame

These foods, on the other hand, have earned high GI ratings:

- Breads: Whole wheat bread, cornbread, all baked goods made with white flour
- Cereals: Old-fashioned oats, corn and most corn products, some rice products, millet, some dry cereals
- Pastas: All thick shapes, including ziti, penne, and rigatoni

- Fruits: Watermelon, raisins, pineapple, cantaloupe, very ripe bananas
- Vegetables: Parsnips; potatoes, including baked russet potatoes, french fries, fresh mashed potatoes, and especially instant mashed potatoes; corn; beets; carrots
- Snacks: Corn chips, tortilla chips, pretzels, rice cakes
- Miscellaneous: Foods sweetened with a lot of sugar, honey, molasses, corn syrup, glucose, or dextrose

As a general rule, choosing foods from the low end of the glycemic index can help maintain healthy blood sugar and melt away body fat to boot. But this doesn't mean you should judge a food solely by its GI. Take oatmeal as an example. It has a GI of 59, but it also is a great source of soluble fiber. You'll benefit more from eating it than avoiding it. Not so with a chocolate bar. Sure, its GI is just 49. But it packs so many calories and so much saturated fat that indulging too many of them could sabotage your weight-loss efforts.

When deciding whether or not to eat a particular food, you really ought to consider its GI in the context of its overall nutritional value. Whole wheat bread and white bread may have similar GIs, but whole wheat is the better choice because it contains extra fiber, among other key nutrients. Similarly, brown rice and whole wheat pastas are more nutritious than white rice and pastas.

If you decide to eat a food that has a high GI, your best bet is to pair it with a food that has either a low GI or more protein or fat. This helps blunt the effect

HOW SWEET IT IS

A food's sweetness doesn't necessarily correlate to its effects on blood sugar. What really matters is the size of the food's sugar molecules, which you can't determine without a powerful microscope.

Also important is ripeness and preparation. If a food is very ripe, or if it has been processed or cooked, it is partially "digested." So its simple sugars will reach your bloodstream more quickly. In general, a food will have a lower glycemic index when raw than when cooked.

on your blood sugar. For instance, you could balance the high GI of oatmeal with the low GI of milk and/or nuts.

The point is, never ban a food from your diet simply because it earned a high GI. Variety, moderation, and balance are the cornerstones of a sensible eating plan. Occasional indulgences are important, too.

IT'S ALL ABOUT INSULIN

The trouble with eating a steady diet of foods from the high end of the glycemic index is the effect on insulin, a hormone that's beneficial in moderation but not in excess. You see, when your body breaks down carbohydrates into glucose, your pancreas responds by releasing insulin. The job of insulin is to grab glucose from the bloodstream and usher it into cells. There, glucose gets turned into energy or—if a cell already has satisfied its energy requirements—into fat.

Every time you eat a food with a high GI, the resulting rise in blood sugar triggers a corresponding rise in insulin. Researchers believe that repeated spikes in insulin levels could increase the risk of diabetes, as well as heart disease and cancer.

Your body has a very precise mechanism for regulating the amount of glucose that moves into cells and the amount that stays in your bloodstream. Building your diet around quickly absorbed carbohydrates—those with high GIs—can disrupt this mechanism. By eating slowly absorbed carbs in balance with lean proteins and healthy fats, you can stabilize your blood sugar and shed those unwanted pounds.

Keep in mind that by choosing unrefined carbohydrates, you get more fiber, which further slows the breakdown of carbs into glucose. This prevents the production of excess insulin, along with sudden or significant drops in blood sugar. As a result, you don't feel as hungry—and you're less likely to experience cravings for sweets.

LOW-CARB Q&A

Scientific research and clinical observations provide convincing proof that a low-carb eating plan is a viable option for those who want to take control of their diabetes and their waistlines. Understandably, you still may have some concerns, given the persistent criticism of the low-carb approach. Perhaps the following Q&A, addressing the most common questions raised by skeptics of low-carb diets, will provide some guidance as you mull over whether to try our plan. (Remember, though, to consult your doctor or a nutritionist before making any changes in your current diet.)

Q: DOES RESTRICTING CARBOHYDRATES CAUSE FATIGUE?

A: Not likely. Some folks have reported a decline in energy for up to three days after switching to a low-carb eating plan. This could be a symptom of withdrawal from refined carbohydrates, which provide an energizing boost to blood sugar—usually followed by a fatigue-inducing plunge. On this plan, you'll get plenty of energy from unrefined carbohydrates, as well as from proteins and fats. And because unrefined carbs break down into glucose more slowly, your blood sugar levels will remain steady.

Q: WILL EATING MORE PROTEINS AND FEWER CARBOHYDRATES DAMAGE MY KIDNEYS?

A: If you've never had kidney trouble, you probably don't need to worry about warnings that eating more protein and fewer carbohydrates will wear out your kidneys. In fact, no research has confirmed this purported risk, even in people who consume three times the recommended amount of protein.

That said, if you already have kidney disease, please be careful about increasing your protein intake. Too much protein could overwhelm weakened kidneys, causing serious long-term damage.

Not sure about your kidney function? Talk with

your doctor about appropriate testing before you change your diet.

Q: WON'T EATING MORE FAT RAISE MY CHOLESTEROL AND TRIGLYCERIDES, FURTHER INCREASING MY RISK OF HEART DISEASE?

A: For years, we heard that eating any kind of fat was unhealthy for the heart. Now we know that saturated fat is the real culprit. Research has shown that people who regularly eat foods rich in monounsaturated and polyunsaturated fats while cutting back on carbohydrates actually lower their total cholesterol. What's more, those who eat fewer carbs have reported rises in beneficial HDL cholesterol and declines in triglycerides.

One possible explanation centers on the relationship between insulin and triglycerides. On a high-carbohydrate diet, your body needs a lot of insulin to metabolize the extra carbs. And as insulin rises, so do triglycerides. To lower triglycerides, then, you want to keep a lid on insulin. A good way to do that is to trim your carbohydrate intake. The bottom line is, a low-carb eating plan could reduce heart disease risk because it whittles away at insulin and triglyceride levels.

Q: DOES CUTTING BACK ON CARBOHYDRATES WHILE INCREASING PROTEINS AND FATS AFFECT EVERYONE'S BLOOD LIPIDS IN THE SAME WAY?

A: The vast majority of people who follow a sensible low-carb eating plan experience dramatic reductions in triglycerides and significant increases in HDL cholesterol. For a small percentage of the population, even the modest rise in dietary fat that's typical of a low-carb approach may cause unhealthy changes in blood lipids. If you have a history of high cholesterol and triglycerides, check with your doctor before making any dietary changes. Schedule a blood workup at the eight-week mark, so you and your doctor can see how your new diet is affecting your blood lipid profile.

Q: WILL EATING MORE PROTEIN ELEVATE MY RISK OF HEART DISEASE?

A: The latest evidence suggests otherwise. In a study at the Harvard School of Public Health, researchers examined the health status of 80,082 women between ages 34 and 59 with no prior indications of heart disease. After controlling for all other risk factors, the researchers determined that both animal and plant proteins helped lower heart disease risk. This held true regardless of whether the women followed a low-fat or high-fat diet. The researchers concluded that replacing refined carbohydrates with proteins actually may be good for the heart.

Q: HOW WILL EATING FEWER CARBOHYDRATES AND MORE PROTEINS AFFECT MY BONE HEALTH?

A: When you increase your protein intake, your blood becomes more acidic. Your body responds by releasing calcium from your bones. This helps restore your blood's pH to a more alkaline state, but at the expense of your calcium stores. Over time, it may set the stage for osteoporosis.

You can help preserve your calcium supply, and your bone health, just by eating lots of vegetables. They help tip the pH scale toward alkaline, so calcium won't have to do the job.

Keep in mind, though, that too little protein—a common problem when following a low-fat diet—can be just as harmful to your bones as too much. For the eating plan presented here, we've set an upper limit on protein intake and provided for plenty of bone-friendly calcium sources like cheeses, leafy greens, salmon, sardines, almonds, Brazil nuts, and calcium-fortified soy products. For insurance, you may want to take a high-quality multivitamin, since so many nutrients besides calcium contribute to bone health. They include magnesium, vitamin D, vitamin C, vitamin K, zinc, boron, lysine, potassium, and silicon.

Q: I'VE HEARD THAT YOU CAN EAT MORE MEAT ON A LOW-CARBOHYDRATE DIET. BUT WHAT ABOUT RESEARCH LINKING MEAT CONSUMPTION TO A HIGHER CANCER RISK?

A: We've seen those same studies. The fact is, scientists still are trying to figure out what does and doesn't cause cancer. In terms of diet, here's what they know so far:

- Toxins that may contribute to cancer are stored in fat.
- Nitrates and nitrites—usually found in smoked, cured, or pickled meats or fish—form nitrosamines, compounds that have been linked to cancer.

- Blackened or charred meats, fish, or poultry contain substances known to play a role in cancer.
- The fatty portions of meat may contain estrogens that contribute to estrogen-dominance-type cancers.

While all these are legitimate concerns, you can take steps to neutralize their impact. For example, eating lots of fruits and vegetables supplies a host of antioxidants that help protect against carcinogens. Whole foods in general supply an assortment of nutrients that support your liver, your body's built-in detoxification system.

Remember, too, that while you may be eating more protein, that doesn't necessarily mean more meat. You can get plenty of protein from beans, nuts, and other plant sources.

Q: WHAT ABOUT OTHER REPORTED "SIDE EFFECTS" OF A LOW-CARBOHYDRATE EATING PLAN, LIKE BAD BREATH AND CONSTIPATION?

A: The so-called ketone breath often associated with low-carbohydrate diets should not be a problem on this eating plan because it does not advocate the sort of severe carb restriction that triggers ketosis. And with all the fiber from vegetables, fruits, legumes, and whole grains, you're unlikely to experience constipation. On the contrary, you may notice improved regularity.

EATING THE SMART LOW-CARB WAY

To help put the principles of low-carbohydrate eating into practice, we've created a sample seven-day menu plan using a number of recipes from Chapter 9, as well as a variety of common foods. Each day's menu supplies 125 grams of carbohydrates, on average. You can choose from three different calorie ranges, based on your body's energy needs.

To determine your ideal calorie intake, first take a look at the following chart and pick the activity factor that best describes your fitness level.

If You Are A . . .	Your Activity Factor Is . . .
Sedentary woman	12
Sedentary man	14
Active woman	15
Active man	17
Very active woman	18
Very active man	20

As a point of reference, "sedentary" means that you work out no more than once a week and your lifestyle involves mostly sitting, standing, or light walking. "Active" describes a lifestyle that is more physically demanding than light walking (such as full-time housecleaning or construction work) or that includes regular aerobic exercise—45 to 60 minutes three days a week. To qualify as "very active," you must work out for at least 45 minutes at least four times a week.

Once you've decided on your activity factor, multiply that figure by your weight in pounds. The result

LOW-CARB, RESTAURANT-STYLE

Planning to eat out? Don't leave your low-carbohydrate diet at home. Since most restaurant entrées emphasize proteins rather than carbs, you shouldn't have to look too hard to find something that suits your dietary guidelines—and appeals to your tastebuds.

Just pay careful attention when reading the menu. Certain terms may suggest a higher carbohydrate content than you really want. All of the following are red flags:

- à la mode
- barbecued
- breaded
- creamed
- crispy
- crust
- fruited
- glazed
- gravy
- honey-baked
- loaf
- parmigiana
- pot pie
- stuffed
- stuffing
- sweet and sour
- tetrazzini

If you're unsure about the preparation of a dish, don't hesitate to ask questions or request substitutions. If bread comes with your meal, remember that an average-size dinner roll equals roughly two starch servings. That's not to discourage you from eating it. As long as it's just an occasional indulgence, it won't have any long-lasting implications for your blood sugar or your waistline.

is the number of calories necessary to maintain your current weight. If you want to slim down, simply reduce your calorie intake by 500 to 1,000 per day. You'll take off a safe and healthy one to two pounds per week.

One final reminder: Please check with your doctor before making any dietary changes, especially if you have diabetes. Then you're set to give this menu plan a test run. In just seven days, you should see improvement in your blood sugar levels—and on the scale!

DAY 1

Menu	Calories		
	1,500–1,800	1,800–2,200	2,200–2,500
Breakfast			
Fried Eggs with Vinegar (page 135)	1 serving	1 serving	1 serving
Whole grain bread	1 slice	1 slice	1 slice
Butter	1 tsp	1 tsp	2 tsp
Fat-free milk	½ cup	½ cup	½ cup
Apple juice	½ cup	½ cup	½ cup
Snack			
Nectarine or pear	1	1	1
Lunch			
Grilled chicken tenders,	4 oz	5 oz	6 oz
brushed with Italian dressing	1 tsp	1 Tbsp	1 Tbsp
Salad made with			
Red leaf lettuce	1 cup	1 cup	1 cup
Carrots, shredded	¼ cup	¼ cup	¼ cup
Cucumber, sliced	½ cup	½ cup	½ cup
Italian dressing	2 tsp	2 Tbsp	2 Tbsp

Snack			
Walnuts	1 oz	1 oz	1 oz
Dinner			
London broil	4 oz	5 oz	7 oz
Spanish-Style Green Beans (page 159)	1 serving	1 serving	1 serving
Couscous	½ cup	½ cup	½ cup
Snack			
Orange-Walnut Biscotti (page 162)	2 cookies	2 cookies	2 cookies
Total calories (approx.)	**1,640**	**1,880**	**2,240**
Total carbs (g)	**125**	**125**	**125**

DAY 2

Menu	**Calories**		
	1,500–1,800	1,800–2,200	2,200–2,500
Breakfast			
Cherry Cream of Rye Cereal (page 138)	1 serving	1 serving	1 serving
Fat-free milk	½ cup	½ cup	½ cup
Turkey sausage	1 oz	1 oz	1 oz
Snack			
Apple	1	1	1
Lunch			
Sandwich made with Tuna	3 oz	4 oz	5 oz
Celery, chopped	¼ cup	¼ cup	¼ cup
Onion, chopped	¼ cup	¼ cup	¼ cup
Mayonnaise, reduced-fat	2 Tbsp	¼ cup	¼ cup

Green olives	10 small	10 small	10 small
Green leaf lettuce, torn	1 cup	1 cup	1 cup
Sourdough bread	1 slice	1 slice	1 slice
Snack			
Pecans	1 oz	1 oz	1½ oz
Dinner			
Pork Chops Baked with Cabbage and Cream (page 150)	1 serving	1 serving	1½ servings
Steamed butternut squash	½ cup	½ cup	½ cup
Snack			
Pumpernickel bread	1 slice	1 slice	½ slice
Swiss cheese, reduced-fat	1 oz	2 oz	2 oz
Butter	1 tsp	2 tsp	2 tsp
Total calories (approx.)	**1,670**	**1,960**	**2,240**
Total carbs (g)	**127**	**127**	**127**

DAY 3

Menu	**Calories**		
	1,500–1,800	1,800–2,200	2,200–2,500
Breakfast			
Scrambled egg	1	2	2
Rye toast	1 slice	1 slice	1 slice
Butter	1 tsp	2 tsp	2 tsp
Orange juice	½ cup	½ cup	½ cup
Fat-free milk	½ cup	½ cup	½ cup
Snack			
Kiwifruit	1	1	1

Lunch			
Salad made with	½ cup	½ cup	½ cup
Lentils, cooked			
Turkey breast, cooked and cubed	3 oz	4 oz	5 oz
Carrots, sliced	½ cup	½ cup	½ cup
Peppers, chopped	½ cup	½ cup	½ cup
Peas, cooked	¼ cup	¼ cup	½ cup
Olive oil	2 tsp	1 Tbsp	4 tsp
Cheddar cheese	½ oz	½ oz	1 oz
Snack			
Brazil nuts	1 oz	1 oz	1 oz
Dinner			
Stir-Fried Chicken and Broccoli (page 151)	1 serving (4 oz chicken)	1 serving (5 oz chicken)	1 serving (7 oz chicken)
Snack			
Pecan Muffins (page 139)	1	1	1
Butter	1 tsp	2 tsp	2 tsp
Total calories (approx.)	**1,590**	**1,960**	**2,240**
Total carbs (g)	**123**	**123**	**123**

DAY 4

Menu	**Calories**		
	1,500–1,800	1,800–2,200	2,200–2,500
Breakfast			
Pecan Muffins (page 139)	1	1	1
Cottage cheese	2 Tbsp	6 Tbsp	6 Tbsp
Peach	1	1	1
Fat-free milk	½ cup	½ cup	½ cup

Snack			
Grapefruit	½	½	½
Lunch			
Sandwich made with Rice cakes	2	2	2
Sardines, boneless, skinless	4 oz	5 oz	6 oz
Cream cheese	2 Tbsp	2 Tbsp	3 Tbsp
Tomato	2 slices	2 slices	2 slices
Zucchini, sticks	½ cup	½ cup	½ cup
Snack			
Almonds	1 oz	1 oz	1 oz
Dinner			
Lamb chop,	4 oz	5 oz	7 oz
baked with garlic powder	⅛ tsp	⅛ tsp	¼ tsp
Mint leaves, chopped	2 tsp	1 Tbsp	1 Tbsp
Barley, cooked	½ cup	½ cup	½ cup
Stewed tomatoes	1 cup	1 cup	1 cup
Green beans,	½ cup	½ cup	½ cup
sautéed in olive oil	2 tsp	3 tsp	4 tsp
Snack			
Whole wheat bread	1 slice	1 slice	1 slice
Butter	1 tsp	2 tsp	2 tsp
Chicken, sliced	1 oz	2 oz	2 oz
Total calories (approx.)	**1,700**	**1,950**	**2,210**
Total carbs (g)	**122**	**122**	**122**

DAY 5

Menu	Calories		
	1,500–1,800	1,800–2,200	2,200–2,500
Breakfast			
Sweet potato,	½ cup	½ cup	½ cup
cooked and topped with walnut oil or canola oil	½ tsp	1 tsp	1 tsp
Walnuts, chopped	1 oz	1 oz	1 oz
Coconut, shredded	1 Tbsp	2 Tbsp	2 Tbsp
Pineapple, crushed	¼ cup	¼ cup	¼ cup
Chicken breast, cooked	—	2 oz	3 oz
Fat-free milk	½ cup	½ cup	½ cup
Snack			
Pear	½	½	½
Lunch			
Salad made with Spinach	2 cups	2 cups	2 cups
Chickpeas	½ cup	½ cup	½ cup
Egg, hard-cooked	1	2	2
Ham, boiled	—	—	2 oz
Artichoke hearts	½ cup	½ cup	½ cup
Olive oil	2 tsp	3 tsp	5 tsp
Lemon juice	1 Tbsp	1 Tbsp	1 Tbsp + 2 tsp
Whole wheat pita	½	½	½
Snack			
Monterey Jack cheese	2 oz	2 oz	2 oz

Dinner

Breaded Baked Cod with Tartar Sauce (page 153)	1 serving	1 serving	1½ servings
Red cabbage,	½ cup	½ cup	½ cup
sautéed in sesame oil	1 tsp	2 tsp	1 tsp
Yellow squash, steamed	½ cup	½ cup	½ cup
Butter	1 tsp	1 tsp	1 tsp
Cantaloupe Sorbet (page 165)	1 serving	1 serving	1 serving

Snack

Popcorn, air-popped	3 cups	3 cups	1½ cups
Butter	1 tsp	2 tsp	2 tsp
Monterey Jack cheese	2 oz	2 oz	2 oz
Total calories (approx.)	**1,640**	**1,980**	**2,310**
Total carbs (g)	**124**	**124**	**124**

DAY 6

Menu	**Calories**		
	1,500–1,800	1,800–2,200	2,200–2,500
Breakfast			
Cottage cheese	¼ cup	½ cup	¾ cup
Blueberries	¾ cup	¾ cup	¾ cup
Cinnamon	Pinch	Pinch	Pinch
Bacon, nitrate-free, cooked	1 slice	2 slices	2 slices
Snack			
Grapes, red	15 small	15 small	15 small
Lunch			
Hamburger, lean	4 oz	5 oz	6 oz
Hamburger bun, whole wheat	½	½	½
Leaf lettuce	1 leaf	1 leaf	1 leaf

Tomato	1 slice	1 slice	1 slice
Onion, sliced	1 slice	1 slice	1 slice
Mustard	1 tsp	1 tsp	1 tsp
Mayonnaise	2 tsp	3 tsp	3 tsp
French fries	10 small	10 small	10 small
Olives, green	—	5 small	10 small
Snack			
Hazelnuts	1 oz	1 oz	1 oz
Cheddar, reduced-fat	—	1½ oz	1½ oz
Dinner			
Mushroom and Kasha Soup (page 141)	1 serving	1 serving	1 serving
Turkey breast, cooked	4 oz	5 oz	7 oz
Carrots, baby, cooked	½ cup	½ cup	½ cup
Peas, cooked	¼ cup	¼ cup	¼ cup
Olive oil	1 tsp	2 tsp	2 tsp
Snack			
Peanut Butter Cookies (page 161)	1 cookie	1 cookie	1 cookie
Fat-free milk	½ cup	½ cup	½ cup
Total calories (approx.)	**1,570**	**1,890**	**2,230**
Total carbs (g)	**125**	**125**	**125**

DAY 7

Menu Calories Levels	1,500–1,800	1,800–2,200	2,200–2,500
Breakfast			
Bran cereal, flaked	½ cup	½ cup	½ cup
Fat-free milk	½ cup	½ cup	½ cup
Banana	½	½	½
Cottage cheese	½ cup	½ cup	½ cup

Snack			
Cherries, large	10	10	10
Protein bar (16 g protein, 2 g carb)	—	¾ bar	¾ bar
Lunch			
Sausage, Egg, and Vegetable Casserole (page 155)	1 serving	1 serving	2 servings
Spinach, steamed	½ cup	½ cup	½ cup
Whole wheat bread	1 slice	1 slice	1 slice
Snack			
Almonds	1 oz	1 oz	1 oz
Swiss cheese, reduced-fat	—	2 oz	2 oz
Dinner			
Scallops in Tarragon Cream (page 154)	1 serving	1 serving	1 serving
Asparagus, steamed	½ cup	½ cup	½ cup
Tomato, broiled	1 large	1 large	—
Brown rice, cooked	½ cup	½ cup	½ cup
Butter	—	1 tsp	1 tsp
Snack			
Gingerbread Cake with Peach Whipped Cream (page 163)	1 serving	1 serving	1 serving
Total calories (approx.)	**1,530**	**1,950**	**2,350**
Total carbs (g)	**128**	**128**	**131**

CHAPTER NINE

Low-Carb Meals That Heal

All of the science in support of a low-carbohydrate approach to weight loss and blood sugar control means little if it doesn't allow for one very important element of success: fabulous-tasting food. In short, no one will stick with an eating plan if they don't enjoy what they're eating.

That's why we've assembled this collection of easy but oh-so-good recipes to tempt your tastebuds without blowing your carbohydrate budget. Several of these dishes are featured in the menu plan presented in Chapter 8. You can substitute as you wish; just remember that doing so will affect your total calorie and carbohydrate intakes for the day.

While most of the recipes fall in the low to moderate range for carbohydrates, a few contain more carbs than you might expect (30-plus grams per serving). You may want to save these foods for a once-in-a-while splurge—say, every other week. Such periodic indulgences are important. They add variety to your eating plan, so sticking with it is easier in the long run.

You also will notice that some recipes are higher in fat, supplying upward of 15 grams per serving. Don't be scared off. Actually, if you want to lose weight, you should eat at least a little bit of fat. The reason: Fat creates a feeling of fullness, so you're less inclined to overeat. Much of the fat in these recipes is of the healthier monounsaturated or polyunsaturated variety. Saturated fat is kept to a minimum.

In addition to a complete nutritional analysis, every recipe comes with a breakdown of its diet exchanges. Some people like to use the diet exchanges to track how much they've eaten across six core food groups: milk (dairy products), vegetable, fruit, bread (starch), meat (protein foods), and fat. The figure preceding each food group reflects the total number of servings provided by the recipe. The diet exchanges can help ensure that you're making healthy, balanced food choices within the context of your overall eating plan.

That said, try not to get too hung up on tallying diet exchanges—or fat or carbohydrates, for that matter. You should enjoy your food, not obsess over it. Anything in moderation has its place in a sensible eating plan.

NOT YOUR USUAL BREAKFAST FARE

Many people say that they either skip breakfast or eat the same thing every morning. Neither is the healthiest or most energizing way to start the day. In fact, the latest research suggests that breakfast may be the best time to eat carbohydrates, since your body is more receptive to the insulin rush produced by carb-rich foods. If you need some enticement to the breakfast table, or if you just need a change of pace, try these delectable dishes.

Fried Eggs with Vinegar

206 calories, 1 g carbs

2 tablespoons butter

8 large eggs

1 teaspoon salt

¼ teaspoon ground black pepper

⅛ teaspoon dried marjoram or basil

4 teaspoons red wine vinegar

1 teaspoon chopped parsley (optional)

Melt 1 tablespoon of the butter in a large nonstick skillet over medium-low heat. Add the eggs and sprinkle with the salt, pepper, and marjoram or basil. Work in batches if necessary. Cover and cook until the whites are set and the yolks are almost set, 3 to 5 minutes. (For steam-basted eggs, add 1 teaspoon water to the pan and cover with a lid.)

Remove to plates. Place the skillet over low heat and add the remaining 1 tablespoon butter. Cook until the butter turns light brown, 1 to 2 minutes. Add the vinegar. Pour the vinegar mixture over the eggs. Sprinkle with the parsley (if using). Serve hot.

Makes 4 servings

Per serving: 206 calories, 13 g protein, 1 g carbohydrates, 16 g fat, 7 g saturated fat, 440 mg cholesterol, 764 mg sodium, 0 g fiber

Diet exchanges: 0 milk, 0 vegetable, 0 fruit, 0 bread, 2 meat, 2½ fat

Time-savers: Cook the eggs 1 to 2 days ahead and keep them in the refrigerator in a covered container for a speedy breakfast or brown-bag lunch. Reheat in a 350°F oven for 8 to 10 minutes. Or serve at room temperature in a sandwich with sprouts and sliced cheese.

Whole Grain Crepes with Banana and Kiwifruit

215 calories, 34 g carbs

Crepes

1 cup whole grain pastry flour
¼ teaspoon salt
1 egg
1 cup + 3 tablespoons unsweetened soy milk or whole milk
1½ teaspoons vanilla extract
2 teaspoons butter
1–2 tablespoons water

Filling

2 cups plain yogurt
1 banana, cut into 16 diagonal slices
2 kiwifruit, peeled, cut in half lengthwise, and sliced
2 teaspoons lime juice (optional)
½ teaspoon ground cinnamon

To make the crepes: In a large bowl, combine the flour and salt.

In a small bowl, beat the egg, then stir in the milk and vanilla. Pour into the flour and mix well.

Melt ½ teaspoon of the butter in an 8" nonstick skillet over medium heat. Pour 3 tablespoons of batter into the skillet and tilt the skillet to coat the bottom in a thin layer. If the batter seems too thick, add 1 to 2 tablespoons water.

Cook the first side until nicely browned, about 2 minutes. Using a spatula, turn the crepe and cook the second side for 1 to 2 minutes (the second side will look spotty). Slide the crepe onto a plate and cover with foil to keep warm.

Continue making crepes in the same fashion, buttering the pan again after every second crepe, until all the butter and batter are used.

To make the filling and assemble: Place a crepe on a serving plate, attractive side down, and spread with 1 tablespoon of the yogurt. Arrange 2 banana slices and a quarter of a kiwifruit in strips one-third of the way from one edge. Sprinkle with ¼ teaspoon of the lime juice and a pinch of the cinnamon, and roll up. Continue assembling the remaining crepes.

Makes 4 servings (eight 6" to 7" crepes)

Per serving: 215 calories, 8 g protein, 34 g carbohydrates, 6 g fat, 3 g saturated fat, 62 mg cholesterol, 198 mg sodium, 6 g fiber

Diet exchanges: ½ milk, 0 vegetable, 1 fruit, 1 bread, 0 meat, 1 fat

Oatmeal with Ricotta, Fruit, and Nuts

184 calories, 30 g carbs

2 cups apple cider
2 cups water
2 cups rolled oats
⅛ teaspoon salt
½ teaspoon ground cinnamon
¼ cup (2 ounces) ricotta cheese
1 large peach or plum (4 ounces), chopped

2 tablespoons sunflower seeds or toasted almonds, chopped

Combine the cider, water, oats, and salt in a medium saucepan. Bring to a boil over medium heat. Reduce the heat to low. Cook, uncovered, until thick and creamy, stirring occasionally, 3 to 5 minutes.

Spoon into bowls and sprinkle with the cinnamon. Top with the ricotta, peach or plum, and nuts or seeds. Serve hot.

Makes 6 servings

Per serving: 184 calories, 6 g protein, 30 g carbohydrates, 4 g fat, 1 g saturated fat, 5 mg cholesterol, 81 mg sodium, 4 g fiber

Diet exchanges: 0 milk, 0 vegetable, 1 fruit, 1 bread, ½ meat, ½ fat

Flavor tips: For chewier oatmeal, bring the cider, water, and salt to a boil, then stir in the oats. For sweeter oatmeal, drizzle each serving with 1 to 2 teaspoons low-calorie maple syrup.

Cherry Cream of Rye Cereal

208 calories, 45 g carbs

1 ¼ cups water
1 ¼ cups apple cider
¼ teaspoon salt
1 cup cream of rye cereal
1 ¼ tablespoons cherry fruit spread
⅛ teaspoon ground nutmeg
⅛ teaspoon ground cardamom
1 ½ tablespoons chopped hazelnuts (optional)

Combine the water, cider, and salt in a saucepan and bring to a boil over medium heat. Stir in the cereal and reduce the heat to low. Cook, uncovered, until thick, stirring occasionally, 3 to 5 minutes. Remove from the heat and stir in the fruit spread.

Spoon into bowls and sprinkle with the nutmeg, cardamom, and hazelnuts (if using). Serve hot.

Makes 4 servings (3 cups)

Per serving: 208 calories, 4 g protein, 45 g carbohydrates, 1 g fat, 0 g saturated fat, 0 mg cholesterol, 168 mg sodium, 6 g fiber

Diet exchanges: 0 milk, 0 vegetable, 1 fruit, 2 bread, 0 meat, 0 fat

Pecan Muffins

218 calories, 20 g carbs

1½ cups whole grain pastry flour
¼ cup soy flour
2½ teaspoons baking powder
½ teaspoon salt
½ teaspoon ground nutmeg
½ cup toasted pecans, chopped
½ cup vegetable oil
½ cup apricot or peach fruit spread
2 large eggs, lightly beaten
1½ teaspoons vanilla extract
⅛ teaspoon liquid stevia (a natural sweetener)

Place a rack in the middle position in the oven and preheat the oven to 375°F. Coat a 12-cup muffin pan with cooking spray or line with paper cups.

In a large bowl, whisk together the pastry flour, soy flour, baking powder, salt, nutmeg, and pecans.

In a small bowl, combine the oil, fruit spread, eggs, vanilla, and stevia. Add to the flour mixture and stir just until the dry ingredients are moistened.

Spoon into the prepared muffin cups until ¾ full. Bake 12 to 14 minutes, until a toothpick inserted in the center of a muffin comes out clean. Serve warm.

Makes 12 muffins

Per serving: 218 calories, 4 g protein, 20 g carbohydrates, 12 g fat, 1 g saturated fat, 35 mg cholesterol, 193 mg sodium, 3 g fiber

Diet exchanges: 0 milk, 0 vegetable, 0 fruit, 1 bread, ½ meat, 2½ fat

Time-savers: Make a double batch and cut preparation time in half. To store, let the muffins cool, then wrap them individually and place in a self-sealing bag. Keep for up to 2 days in the refrigerator or 2 months in the freezer. Thaw the muffins at room temperature and reheat on a baking sheet at 350°F for 5 to 10 minutes.

LUNCHES THAT SATISFY

Say goodbye to the fast-food drive-through! Even if you don't have much time for lunch, you still can enjoy a tasty low-carb meal. You may need to do a little advance preparation, but it's worth the effort.

One option is to double the recipe that's on the menu for dinner, then store each extra serving in a microwaveable container in the refrigerator. Come lunchtime the next day, just reheat, and you're ready to eat.

If you're fond of salads, pick up some prepared greens at the supermarket. For protein, add chickpeas or chunks of chicken, turkey, or hard-cooked eggs. Then get creative with toppings like Parmesan cheese, sunflower seeds, olives, and real bacon bits.

Want more choices? All of the following are perfect for lunch-on-the-go.

Mushroom and Kasha Soup

112 calories, 11 g carbs

½ cup kasha (buckwheat groats)
2 tablespoons olive oil
20 ounces mushrooms, coarsely chopped
½ onion, finely chopped
1 carrot, finely chopped
1½ celery ribs, finely chopped
½ red bell pepper, finely chopped
½ teaspoon ground black pepper
2¼ cans (14½ ounces each) chicken or vegetable broth
1 teaspoon dried dill or thyme
1 bay leaf

Toast the kasha in a soup pot over medium heat for 2 to 3 minutes, stirring frequently. Remove to a bowl.

Heat the oil in the same pot over medium-low heat. Stir in the mushrooms, onion, carrot, celery, bell pepper, and black pepper. Cover and cook, stirring occasionally, for 8 to 10 minutes.

Stir in the kasha and broth. Bring to a simmer and add the dill or thyme and the bay leaf. Partially cover, and cook until the kasha is tender, about 10 minutes. Remove the bay leaf before serving.

Makes 6 servings

Per serving: 112 calories, 6 g protein, 11 g carbohydrates, 6 g fat, 1 g saturated fat, 0 mg cholesterol, 687 mg sodium, 3 g fiber

Diet exchanges: 0 milk, 1½ vegetable, 0 fruit, ½ bread, 0 meat, 1 fat

Flavor tips: Serve sprinkled with chopped scallions. For a vegetarian stew, cook with only 1 cup vegetable broth.

White Bean Soup with Sausage

218 calories, 17 g carbs

1 tablespoon + 1 teaspoon olive oil

½ pound sweet Italian sausage, casing removed, broken into 1" pieces

½ large onion, chopped

3 celery ribs, chopped

2½ cups (8 ounces) chopped green or red cabbage

1 cup (8 ounces) dried white beans, soaked overnight and drained

4–5 cans (14 ½ ounces each) reduced-sodium chicken broth

1 can (15 ounces) no-salt-added stewed tomatoes

1 teaspoon dried Italian seasoning

1 large bay leaf

¼ teaspoon ground black pepper

Heat 1 teaspoon of the oil in a soup pot over medium-low heat. Add the sausage and cook, stirring occasionally, just until cooked through, about 5 minutes. Remove to a plate, cover, and refrigerate.

Pour the remaining 1 tablespoon oil into the same pot over medium heat and stir in the onion, celery, and cabbage.

Cook, stirring occasionally, until the vegetables begin to soften, 8 to 10 minutes.

Add the beans, 4 cans of the broth, and the tomatoes to the pot. Bring to a boil and immediately lower the heat, skimming off any froth that comes to the top. Stir in the Italian seasoning and bay leaf. Partially cover, and cook until the beans are tender, 1 ¼ to 1 ½ hours depending on the beans. Add more broth if the soup becomes too thick.

Stir in the sausage and pepper; simmer for 2 minutes. Discard the bay leaf before serving.

Makes 8 servings

Per serving: 218 calories, 12 g protein, 17 g carbohydrates, 13 g fat, 4 g saturated fat, 26 mg cholesterol, 538 mg sodium, 5 g fiber

Diet exchanges: 0 milk, 1 ½ vegetable, 0 fruit, ½ bread, 1 meat, 2 fat

Mexican-Style Summer Squash Soup

86 calories, 9 g carbs

1 ½ tablespoons butter
½ large onion, thinly sliced
4 zucchini and/or yellow squash (24 ounces), chopped
2 garlic cloves, minced
½ large red bell pepper, chopped
¼ cup drained, chopped canned tomatoes
2¼ cans (14½ ounces each) chicken broth
½ teaspoon ground black pepper
½ teaspoon dried oregano
¼ teaspoon ground cumin
1 ½ tablespoons cornmeal

Melt the butter in a medium soup pot over medium heat. Stir in the onion, zucchini or squash, garlic, and bell pepper.

Cook, stirring occasionally, until excess liquid from the squash has evaporated, 8 to 10 minutes.

Stir in the tomatoes and broth. Reduce the heat to low and stir in the black pepper, oregano, and cumin. Cook the soup, uncovered, until the vegetables are tender, about 10 minutes.

Stir in the cornmeal and cook until thickened slightly, 5 minutes.

Makes 6 servings

Per serving: 86 calories, 4 g protein, 9 g carbohydrates, 4 g fat, 2 g saturated fat, 8 mg cholesterol, 694 mg sodium, 3 g fiber

Diet exchanges: 0 milk, 1 vegetable, 0 fruit, ½ bread, 0 meat, ½ fat

Flavor tips: Cook 3 bacon slices in the saucepan until crisp. Drain on a plate lined with paper towel. Use 1½ tablespoons of the drippings in place of the butter to cook the vegetables. Crumble the bacon over each serving. For a thinner soup, omit the cornmeal.

Cincinnati-Style Turkey Chili

306 calories, 29 g carbs

1 tablespoon + 1½ teaspoons vegetable oil
1 large onion, chopped
1 large green bell pepper, chopped
2 garlic cloves, chopped
1⅓ pounds ground turkey
1¾ cups chicken broth
3 tablespoons tomato paste
2–3 tablespoons chili powder
1½ teaspoons dried oregano
1 teaspoon ground coriander

¼ teaspoon salt
½ teaspoon ground cumin
¼ teaspoon ground cinnamon
1 can (15 ounces) red kidney beans (with juice)
6 ounces whole wheat spaghetti, broken into short pieces
½ cup (2 ounces) shredded Monterey Jack or Muenster cheese

Heat the oil in a large, heavy pot over medium heat. Add the onion, bell pepper, and garlic. Cook, stirring occasionally, until the onion starts to brown, 8 to 10 minutes.

Add the turkey and cook, stirring to coarsely crumble until no longer pink, 8 to 10 minutes. Stir in the broth, tomato paste, chili powder, oregano, coriander, salt, cumin, and cinnamon. Bring to a simmer. Partially cover and cook, stirring occasionally, until the meat is tender and the broth is slightly thickened, about 30 minutes.

Meanwhile, pour the beans (with juice) into a microwaveable bowl. Microwave on high power for 1 to 2 minutes or until heated through. Drain and cover to keep warm.

Cook the pasta according to the package directions. Drain and divide among 4 bowls. Ladle the chili over the pasta, top with the beans, and sprinkle with the cheese.

Makes 4 servings

Per serving: 306 calories, 22 g protein, 29 g carbohydrates, 13 g fat, 3 g saturated fat, 66 mg cholesterol, 519 mg sodium, 7 g fiber

Diet exchanges: 0 milk, 1 vegetable, 0 fruit, 1½ bread, 2 meat, 1 fat

Time-saver: The meat mixture will keep in a covered container in the refrigerator for up to 5 days or in the freezer for up to 2 months. To reheat the meat, first thaw in the refrigerator for 12 hours if frozen. Then place in a saucepan set over low heat and cook, stirring frequently, until heated through, about 15 minutes. Cook the pasta and heat the beans right before serving.

Tropical Chicken Salad Sandwiches

380 calories, 18 g carbs

1 container (6 ounces) low-fat piña colada or coconut yogurt
¼ cup light mayonnaise
1 can (8 ounces) crushed pineapple, drained
½ teaspoon poultry seasoning
¼ teaspoon salt
1 pound boneless, skinless cooked chicken breast, chopped
⅔ cup red or white seedless grapes (about 16), halved
1 small celery rib, chopped
1 small apple, chopped (optional)
½ cup sliced toasted almonds
2 tablespoons chopped chives or scallions (optional)
8 large Boston lettuce leaves

In a large bowl, combine the yogurt, mayonnaise, pineapple, poultry seasoning, and salt. Stir in the chicken, grapes, celery, apple (if using), almonds, and chives or scallions (if using).

Arrange the lettuce on a work surface with the rib end closest to you and the "cup" facing up. Divide the salad among the lettuce leaves and roll up into 8 small sandwiches.

Makes 4 servings

Per serving: 380 calories, 41 g protein, 18 g carbohydrates, 16 g fat, 3 g saturated fat, 104 mg cholesterol, 390 mg sodium, 2 g fiber

Diet exchanges: 0 milk, 0 vegetable, 1 fruit, 0 bread, 6 meat, 2½ fat

Tuna Salad in Lettuce Wrappers

222 calories, 2 g carbs

2 cans (6 ounces each) water-packed tuna, drained
¼ cup mayonnaise
1 teaspoon Dijon mustard
1 tablespoon lemon juice
2 tablespoons finely chopped red bell pepper or celery
2 teaspoons capers, drained
2 scallions, thinly sliced
¼ teaspoon salt
⅛ teaspoon ground black pepper
8 large lettuce leaves, such as Boston or leaf

In a bowl, flake the tuna with a fork. Stir in the mayonnaise, mustard, and lemon juice. Stir in the bell pepper or celery, capers, scallions, salt, and pepper.

Arrange the lettuce on a work surface with the rib end closest to you and the "cup" facing up. Spoon the tuna salad onto the leaf near the rib end and roll to enclose.

Makes 4 servings

Per serving: 222 calories, 21 g protein, 2 g carbohydrates, 14 g fat, 3 g saturated fat, 46 mg cholesterol, 621 mg sodium, 1 g fiber

Diet exchanges: 0 milk, ½ vegetable, 0 fruit, 0 bread, 3½ meat, 2 fat

Flavor tips: Substitute canned or cooked salmon or boneless, skinless sardines for the tuna. Add 1 chopped hard-cooked egg and ½ teaspoon dried dill to the salad. You can also add 3 or 4 thin slices of apple or a slice of Swiss or mozzarella cheese to the wrap.

Italian-Style Beef Burgers

252 calories, 2 g carbs

1½ pounds extra-lean ground beef chuck
5 tablespoons (1 ounce) grated Romano cheese
2 tablespoons (1 ounce) pine nuts, toasted and finely chopped
½ teaspoon salt
1 teaspoon dried oregano
¾ teaspoon garlic powder
¼ teaspoon ground black pepper

Place the broiler rack 2" to 3" from the heat source and preheat the broiler.

Place the beef in a large bowl and break into pieces. Add the Romano, nuts, salt, oregano, garlic powder, and pepper. Using a fork, gently combine the beef and seasonings.

Divide the meat into 4 even pieces and gently form into burgers approximately 4" in diameter and 1" thick. Place on a broiling pan, and cook until the top is browned, 4 to 6 minutes. Turn, and cook until done and a meat thermometer registers 160°F for medium, 4 to 6 minutes.

Makes 4 servings

Per serving: 252 calories, 37 g protein, 2 g carbohydrates, 12 g fat, 5 g saturated fat, 98 mg cholesterol, 482 mg sodium, 0 g fiber

Diet exchanges: 0 milk, 0 vegetable, 0 fruit, 0 bread, 5 meat, 1½ fat

DIVINE DINNER IDEAS

Dinner is by far the easiest meal in a low-carb eating plan. Typically, some type of protein food—meat, chicken, or fish—is the star of the plate, with a serving or two of vegetables in supporting roles. Carbohydrates appear sparingly.

Do try to change your protein source from one dinner to the next, to avoid "food fatigue." These recipes will add variety to your eating plan.

London Broil Marinated in Soy Sauce and Mustard

309 calories, 1 g carbs

1 tablespoon dry mustard
4 teaspoons soy sauce
2 teaspoons red wine vinegar
1 teaspoon onion powder
1/4 teaspoon garlic powder
1 tablespoon olive oil
1 top round or sirloin London broil (1 1/2 pounds), 1" thick
1/4 teaspoon salt
1/4 teaspoon ground black pepper

In a small bowl, combine the mustard and soy sauce to make a paste. Stir in the vinegar, onion powder, and garlic powder. Whisk in the olive oil.

Place the beef in a glass baking dish. Pour the mustard mixture over the beef and rub lightly to coat all over. Cover and refrigerate for 2 hours or up to 24 hours. Remove from the refrigerator 15 minutes before cooking.

Place the broiler rack 2" to 3" from the heat source and preheat the broiler. Coat a broiling pan with cooking spray. Transfer the beef to the pan, and sprinkle with the salt and pepper. Broil until the top is browned, 4 to 5 minutes. Turn, and cook the second side until a meat thermometer registers 145°F for medium-rare, 3 to 4 minutes.

Remove to a platter and let rest for 5 minutes. Thinly slice diagonally and serve with the juices on the platter.

Makes 4 servings

Per serving: 309 calories, 36 g protein, 1 g carbohydrates, 17 g fat, 6 g saturated fat, 85 mg cholesterol, 560 mg sodium, 0 g fiber

Diet exchanges: 0 milk, 0 vegetable, 0 fruit, 0 bread, 5 meat, 3 fat

Pork Chops Baked with Cabbage and Cream

463 calories, 12 g carbs

1 small head (1 ½ pounds) green cabbage, cored and finely shredded

4 boneless pork chops (6 ounces each), each ¾" thick

½ teaspoon salt

¼ teaspoon ground black pepper

2 teaspoons olive oil

½ cup half-and-half

1 teaspoon caraway seeds

½ teaspoon sweet Hungarian paprika

1 teaspoon dried marjoram or thyme

½ cup (2 ounces) shredded Swiss cheese

Preheat the oven to 350°F.

Bring a large pot of salted water to a boil over high heat. Add the cabbage and cook until soft, 4 to 5 minutes. Drain in a colander and dry well with paper towels.

Season the meat with ¼ teaspoon of the salt and the pepper. Heat the oil in a large, heavy, oven-safe skillet over high heat. Add the meat and cook just until browned, 1 to 2 minutes. Remove to a plate.

Discard any fat in the skillet and reduce the heat to low. Stir in the cabbage, half-and-half, caraway seeds, paprika, marjoram or thyme, and the remaining ¼ teaspoon salt. Cook and stir until heated through, about 1 minute.

Remove the skillet from the heat and arrange the pork over the cabbage, adding any juices accumulated on the plate. Sprinkle with the cheese. Bake until a meat thermometer registers 160°F for medium-well, about 25 minutes.

Makes 4 servings

Per serving: 463 calories, 53 g protein, 12 g carbohydrates, 20 g fat, 9 g saturated fat, 165 mg cholesterol, 460 mg sodium, 4 g fiber

Diet exchanges: 0 milk, 2½ vegetable, 0 fruit, 0 bread, 7 meat, 3½ fat

Stir-Fried Chicken and Broccoli

321 calories, 18 g carbs

½ cup chicken broth

3 tablespoons Chinese oyster sauce

2 tablespoons orange juice

1 tablespoon + 1½ teaspoons soy sauce

2 cloves garlic, minced

2 teaspoons minced fresh ginger

1 teaspoon sesame oil

¼ teaspoon hot-pepper sauce (optional)

1 tablespoon cornstarch

1 tablespoon + 1½ teaspoons cold water

3 tablespoons vegetable oil
1 pound boneless, skinless chicken breasts, cut into thin strips
1 large bunch (2 pounds) broccoli, cut into small florets
5 scallions, sliced
1 teaspoon toasted sesame seeds (optional)

In a small bowl, combine the broth, oyster sauce, orange juice, soy sauce, garlic, ginger, sesame oil, and hot-pepper sauce (if using).

In a cup, dissolve the cornstarch in the cold water.

Heat the oil in a large wok or skillet over high heat until the oil just starts to smoke. Add the chicken and cook, stirring continually until no longer pink on the surface, about 30 seconds. Stir in the broccoli and cook, stirring continually, until it turns bright green and the chicken is half-cooked, about 2 minutes.

Pour in the broth mixture and cook, stirring frequently, for 2 minutes. Stir in the scallions and cornstarch mixture. Cook, stirring, until the sauce comes to a boil, thickens, and the chicken is cooked through, about 1 minute. Sprinkle with the sesame seeds (if using).

Makes 4 servings

Per serving: 321 calories, 34 g protein, 18 g carbohydrates, 14 g fat, 1 g saturated fat, 66 mg cholesterol, 692 mg sodium, 8 g fiber

Diet exchanges: 0 milk, 3 vegetable, 0 fruit, 0 bread, 4 meat, 2½ fat

Flavor tips: Replace half of the broccoli with ½ bunch sliced bok choy or 2 cups string beans. Replace the chicken with small shrimp or slivered pork.

Breaded Baked Cod with Tartar Sauce

268 calories, 14 g carbs

Tartar Sauce

½ cup reduced-fat mayonnaise
1½ tablespoons lemon juice
1 tablespoon finely chopped dill or sweet pickles
2 teaspoons mustard
2 teaspoons capers, drained and chopped
2 teaspoons chopped parsley (optional)

Fish

2 slices whole wheat bread, torn
2 eggs
1 tablespoon water
1¼ pounds cod or scrod fillet, cut into 1"–1½" pieces
½ teaspoon salt
¼ teaspoon ground black pepper

To make the tartar sauce: In a small bowl, combine the mayonnaise, lemon juice, pickles, mustard, capers, and parsley (if using). Cover and refrigerate.

To make the fish: Preheat the oven to 400°F. Coat a baking sheet with cooking spray.

Place the bread in a food processor and process into fine crumbs. Place in a shallow bowl. In another bowl, beat the eggs with the water.

Season the fish with the salt and pepper. Dip into the eggs, then into the bread crumbs. Place on the prepared baking sheet. Generously coat the breaded fish with cooking spray. Bake until opaque inside, 10 minutes. Serve with the tartar sauce.

Makes 4 servings

Per serving: 268 calories, 30 g protein, 14 g carbohydrates, 10 g fat, 2 g saturated fat, 174 mg cholesterol, 734 mg sodium, 1 g fiber

Diet exchanges: 0 milk, 0 vegetable, 0 fruit, 1 bread, 3½ meat, ½ fat

Time-savers: Cook a few extra pieces of fish, as the leftovers make quick hot or cold meals. Store extra portions in a covered container in the refrigerator for up to 3 days. To reheat, arrange on a baking sheet and bake at 400°F until heated through, 3 to 5 minutes. Or to serve cold, make a sandwich by wrapping the fried fish in lettuce leaves or whole wheat pitas spread with tartar sauce. The tartar sauce can be stored in a covered container in the refrigerator for up to a week.

Scallops in Tarragon Cream

201 calories, 5 g carbs

1 tablespoon butter, softened

1½ pounds fresh or thawed frozen sea scallops, rinsed

1½ teaspoons chopped fresh tarragon or ½ teaspoon dried

¼ teaspoon ground black pepper

¼ cup half-and-half

1 tablespoon Pernod or 2 tablespoons dry sherry (optional)

2 tablespoons lemon juice

1 tablespoon chopped fresh parsley

Melt the butter in a large skillet over medium-high heat. When the butter foams, add the scallops, tarragon, and pepper. Cook for 2 to 3 minutes, stirring constantly.

Stir in the half-and-half, Pernod or sherry (if using), and

lemon juice. Reduce the heat to medium-low and cook until the scallops look opaque throughout and feel slightly springy when lightly pressed, 1 to 2 minutes. Stir in the parsley.

Makes 4 servings

Per serving: 201 calories, 29 g protein, 5 g carbohydrates, 6 g fat, 3 g saturated fat, 71 mg cholesterol, 312 mg sodium, 0 g fiber

Diet exchanges: 0 milk, 0 vegetable, 0 fruit, 0 bread, 4 meat, 1 fat

Flavor tips: Both frozen and fresh scallops can have a briny flavor, so don't season them with salt until you've tasted them. If the sauce in the pan is too thin for your taste, remove the scallops and cook the sauce over medium heat until slightly reduced. Pour over the scallops.

Sausage, Egg, and Vegetable Casserole

352 calories, 7 g carbs

1 pound sweet Italian sausage, casing removed and meat cut into 1" pieces
1 tablespoon + 1½ teaspoons olive oil
½ small head (4 ounces total) escarole, chopped
2 zucchini (8 ounces), thinly sliced
1 red bell pepper, chopped
1 small red onion, thinly sliced
¼ teaspoon salt
¼ teaspoon ground black pepper
7 large eggs, at room temperature
½ cup 2% milk, at room temperature
¼ cup (1 ounce) grated Parmesan cheese

Preheat the oven to 350°F. Coat an 8" × 8" baking dish with cooking spray.

Cook the sausage in a large skillet over medium-high heat until half-cooked, 6 to 8 minutes, stirring occasionally. Spread over the bottom of the prepared dish. Discard the fat in the skillet.

Pour the oil into the same skillet and stir in the escarole, zucchini, bell pepper, onion, salt, and ⅛ teaspoon of the black pepper. Reduce the heat to medium. Cook, stirring occasionally, until the vegetables are tender and the liquid evaporates, 8 to 10 minutes. Let cool for 10 minutes and arrange over the sausage.

Meanwhile, in a large bowl, combine the eggs, milk, cheese, and remaining ⅛ teaspoon black pepper. Pour over the vegetables. Bake until the eggs are set, 40 to 45 minutes. Cut into squares to serve.

Makes 6 servings

Per serving: 352 calories, 23 g protein, 7 g carbohydrates, 26 g fat, 7 g saturated fat, 308 mg cholesterol, 657 mg sodium, 2 g fiber

Diet exchanges: 0 milk, 1 vegetable, 0 fruit, 0 bread, 3 meat, 3½ fat

Flavor tips: Substitute kale, broccoli rabe, or broccoli for the escarole. Replace the pork sausage with chicken or turkey sausage.

Eggplant Parmesan

224 calories, 16 g carbs

2 eggplants (32 ounces total), peeled and sliced lengthwise into slabs ¼" thick

3 tablespoons olive oil

½ teaspoon salt

1 can (15½ ounces) crushed or chopped tomatoes (with juice)

1 tablespoon + 1½ teaspoons tomato paste
1 teaspoon dried basil or 3 large fresh leaves, chopped
½ teaspoon dried rosemary, crumbled
¼ teaspoon ground black pepper
1 cup (4 ounces) shredded mozzarella or Fontina cheese
½ cup (2 ounces) grated Parmesan cheese

Preheat the broiler.

Place the eggplant on a large baking sheet and brush both sides with the oil. Work in batches if necessary. Sprinkle with ¼ teaspoon of the salt. Broil 5" from the heat until just beginning to brown, 2 to 3 minutes per side.

Set the oven temperature to 375°F.

In a saucepan, combine the tomatoes (with juice), tomato paste, basil, and rosemary. Cook over medium-low heat, stirring occasionally, until slightly thickened, about 15 minutes. Season with the remaining ¼ teaspoon salt and the pepper.

Spread a layer of the tomato mixture over the bottom of a 1½-quart baking dish. Add a layer of eggplant and top with another layer of the tomato mixture. Sprinkle with a thin layer of the mozzarella or Fontina and the Parmesan.

Continue making 2 more layers with the remaining eggplant, tomato mixture, and cheeses, ending with a thick layer of cheeses. Bake until bubbling, 25 to 30 minutes. Let rest for 10 minutes before cutting.

Makes 6 servings

Per serving: 224 calories, 11 g protein, 16 g carbohydrates, 14 g fat, 5 g saturated fat, 22 mg cholesterol, 628 mg sodium, 5 g fiber

Diet exchanges: 0 milk, 3 vegetable, 0 fruit, 0 bread, 1 meat, 2 fat

Flavor tips: Substitute ½ cup (2 ounces) shredded Swiss for ½ cup mozzarella cheese. For a smooth sauce, puree the tomatoes in a food mill or food processor. Use the eggplant peeled or unpeeled.

Red Cabbage with Apples

122 calories, 15 g carbs

2 tablespoons rendered bacon fat or walnut oil
6 cups (about ½ small head) shredded red cabbage
⅓ cup apple juice or cider
1 large Granny Smith or other tart apple, peeled and coarsely chopped
2 tablespoons red wine vinegar or other vinegar
¾ teaspoon dried thyme
¼ teaspoon ground allspice
¼ teaspoon salt
⅛ teaspoon ground black pepper

Heat the bacon fat or oil in a Dutch oven or large, deep skillet over medium-low heat. Stir in the cabbage and cook, stirring occasionally, until it begins to wilt, 5 to 6 minutes.

Stir in the apple juice or cider, the apple, vinegar, thyme, and allspice. Cover and cook over low heat until the cabbage is very tender, 25 to 30 minutes, stirring occasionally. Season with the salt and pepper.

Makes 4 servings

Per serving: 122 calories, 2 g protein, 15 g carbohydrates, 7 g fat, 1 g saturated fat, 0 mg cholesterol, 165 mg sodium, 4 g fiber

Diet exchanges: 0 milk, 1 vegetable, ½ fruit, 0 bread, 0 meat, 1½ fat

Time-saver: Make this German-style dish whenever you have a minute. It keeps in a covered container in the refrigerator for up to 5 days. To reheat, place it in a skillet and add 1 to 2 tablespoons water. Cover and cook over low heat, stirring occasionally, until heated through, 3 to 4 minutes.

Spanish-Style Green Beans

162 calories, 13 g carbs

16 ounces green beans, trimmed and cut into 2" lengths
3 tablespoons olive oil
1 onion, chopped
1 small green bell pepper, chopped
1 tomato (4 ounces), peeled, seeded, and coarsely chopped
2 garlic cloves, minced
¼ teaspoon salt
⅛ teaspoon ground black pepper
2–3 tablespoons coarsely chopped, pitted kalamata olives
2 teaspoons drained capers (optional)

Combine the beans, oil, onion, bell pepper, tomato, garlic, salt, and black pepper in a saucepan over medium heat. Cook, stirring, until the vegetables start to sizzle, 2 to 3 minutes.

Reduce the heat to low, cover, and cook, stirring occasionally, until the beans are very tender but not falling apart, 20 to 25 minutes. Stir in the olives and capers (if using) and heat 1 minute. Serve warm, at room temperature, or chilled.

Makes 4 servings

Per serving: 162 calories, 2 g protein, 13 g carbohydrates, 12 g fat, 2 g saturated fat, 0 mg cholesterol, 230 mg sodium, 6 g fiber

Diet exchanges: 0 milk, 2 ½ vegetable, 0 fruit, 0 bread, 0 meat, 2 ½ fat

Bitter Greens with Goat Cheese, Pine Nuts, and Pears

159 calories, 7 g carbs

3 tablespoons (3 ounces) log-type goat cheese
1 tablespoon olive or walnut oil
2–3 tablespoons 2% milk
1 tablespoon lemon juice
⅛ teaspoon salt
⅛ teaspoon ground black pepper
2 large heads Belgian endive, leaves separated and cut into 1" diagonal slices
1 large bunch watercress, chopped
2 tablespoons toasted pine nuts
½ large bosc pear (4 ounces total), cut into ½" cubes

In a blender, combine the cheese, oil, 2 tablespoons of the milk, the lemon juice, salt, and pepper. Process until thickened and creamy, adding up to another tablespoon of milk if too thick.

Place the endive and watercress in a large salad bowl, add the cheese mixture, and toss to combine. Divide among 4 plates. Sprinkle with the nuts and pear.

Makes 4 servings

Per serving: 159 calories, 7 g protein, 7 g carbohydrates, 12 g fat, 5 g saturated fat, 17 mg cholesterol, 214 mg sodium, 2 g fiber

Diet exchanges: 0 milk, 0 vegetable, ½ fruit, 0 bread, 1 meat, 2 fat

Flavor tips: Substitute 4 cups mixed baby spring greens or 1 large bunch arugula for the Belgian endive. Substitute 2 kiwifruits for the pear. Keep the dressing refrigerated in a covered container for up to 5 days. Bring to room temperature before using.

TEMPTING TREATS

To maintain steady blood sugar and prevent unhealthy spikes, many nutrition experts recommend eating at regular intervals throughout the day. So if you're accustomed to the standard three squares—breakfast, lunch, and dinner—you can fill in the gaps with healthy snacks. These will satisfy your urge for something sweet without compromising your commitment to low-carb eating.

Peanut Butter Cookies

94 calories, 7 g carbs

6 tablespoons unsalted butter, softened
½ cup unsweetened smooth peanut butter, at room temperature
¼ cup packed light brown sugar
¼ cup Splenda (a sugar substitute)
1 large egg, at room temperature, lightly beaten
1 teaspoon vanilla extract
1 ¼ cups sifted oat flour
¼ teaspoon baking powder
3 tablespoons salted peanuts, chopped

Place an oven rack in the middle position and preheat the oven to 350°F.

In a large bowl, beat together the butter and peanut butter until very smooth, about 1 minute. Add the brown sugar and Splenda and beat until well-combined and light in color, 1 to 2 minutes.

Gradually beat in the egg and vanilla extract, beating until very smooth and a little fluffy, 1 to 2 minutes. Mix in the flour and baking powder, beating until a moist but cohesive dough forms. Stir in the peanuts.

Drop by tablespoon about 2" apart on nonstick baking sheets. Using the tines of a fork dampened in cold water, flatten each in a cross-hatch pattern until 2" in diameter. Bake until golden brown, 22 to 25 minutes. Remove to a rack to cool.

Makes 24

Per cookie: 94 calories, 3 g protein, 7 g carbohydrates, 7 g fat, 2 g saturated fat, 17 mg cholesterol, 56 mg sodium, 1 g fiber

Diet exchanges: 0 milk, 0 vegetable, 0 fruit, ½ bread, ½ meat, 1 fat

Orange-Walnut Biscotti

76 calories, 8 g carbs

⅔ cup walnuts

¼ cup sugar

1¼ cups whole grain pastry flour

¼ cup cornmeal

1 teaspoon baking powder

¼ teaspoon salt

¼ cup butter, softened

¼ cup Splenda (a sugar substitute)

2 eggs

2 teaspoons grated orange peel

½ teaspoon orange extract

In a food processor, combine the walnuts and 2 tablespoons of the sugar. Process until the walnuts are coarsely ground but not made into a paste. Transfer to a large bowl and add the flour, cornmeal, baking powder, and salt. Stir until combined.

In a large bowl, using an electric mixer, beat the butter, Splenda, and remaining 2 tablespoons sugar until light and fluffy. Beat in the eggs, orange peel, and orange extract. Gradually beat in the flour mixture until smooth and thick.

Divide the dough into two equal-size pieces. Refrigerate for 30 minutes, or until firm.

Preheat the oven to 350°F. Coat a baking sheet with cooking spray.

Shape each piece of dough into a 12"-long log and place both on the prepared baking sheet. Bake for 25 to 30 minutes, or until golden. Remove the logs to wire racks to cool.

Cut each log on a slight diagonal into ½"-thick slices. Place the slices, cut side down, on the baking sheet and bake for 5 minutes. Turn the slices over and bake 5 minutes more, or until dry. Remove to wire racks to cool.

Makes 24

Per biscotto: 76 calories, 2 g protein, 8 g carbohydrates, 5 g fat, 2 g saturated fat, 23 mg cholesterol, 68 mg sodium, 1 g fiber

Diet exchanges: 0 milk, 0 vegetable, 0 fruit, ½ bread, 0 meat, 1 fat

Gingerbread Cake with Peach Whipped Cream

238 calories, 25 g carbs

1½ cups sifted oat flour

¾ cup whole grain pastry flour
2 teaspoons baking powder
1 teaspoon ground ginger
1 teaspoon ground cinnamon
½ teaspoon ground cloves
Pinch of salt
¼ cup light molasses
⅓ cup vegetable oil
1¼ cups hot water
1 teaspoon baking soda
1 large egg + 1 yolk, at room temperature, lightly beaten
¼ teaspoon liquid stevia (a natural sweetener) or ¼ cup Splenda (a sugar substitute)
½ cup heavy cream
3 tablespoons peach fruit spread, at room temperature

Preheat the oven to 350°F. Coat an 8" round cake pan or 8" × 8" baking pan with cooking spray.

In a medium bowl, combine the oat flour, pastry flour, baking powder, ginger, cinnamon, cloves, and salt. In a large bowl, combine the molasses and oil. In a 2-cup glass measure, combine the water and baking soda. Whisk into the molasses-oil mixture.

Gradually whisk the dry ingredients into the molasses mixture. Whisk in the egg, yolk, and stevia or Splenda. Pour into the prepared pan and bake about 30 minutes, until a toothpick inserted in the center comes out clean.

Cool in the pan on a rack for 10 minutes. Remove to the rack and cool completely.

In a large bowl, whip the cream and fruit spread together until firm, but soft, peaks form. Serve wedges of cake topped with a spoonful of the peach cream.

Makes 10 servings

Per serving: 238 calories, 4 g protein, 25 g carbohydrates, 14 g fat, 4 g saturated fat, 59 mg cholesterol, 262 mg sodium, 3 g fiber

Diet exchanges: 0 milk, 0 vegetable, 0 fruit, 1½ bread, 0 meat, 2½ fat

Cantaloupe Sorbet

61 calories, 15 g carbs

4 cups frozen cantaloupe, slightly thawed

1 frozen banana, sliced

¼ cup Splenda (a sugar substitute)

1 tablespoon crème de menthe liqueur (optional)

1 tablespoon lime juice

2 teaspoons grated lime peel

⅛–¼ teaspoon ground cinnamon

In a food processor, combine the cantaloupe, banana, Splenda, liqueur (if using), lime juice, lime peel, and cinnamon. Process until smooth.

Scrape into a shallow metal pan. Cover and freeze for 4 hours or overnight. Using a knife, break the mixture into chunks. Process briefly in a food processor before serving.

Makes 6 servings

Per serving: 61 calories, 1 g protein, 15 g carbohydrates, 0 g fat, 0 g saturated fat, 0 mg cholesterol, 11 mg sodium, 2 g fiber

Diet exchanges: 0 milk, 0 vegetable, 1 fruit, 0 bread, 0 meat, 0 fat

Flavor tips: Frozen cantaloupe saves time in this recipe, but fresh will have more flavor. Use the flesh of 1 small cantaloupe, cut into chunks. For a sweeter sorbet, replace the

Splenda with ¼ cup sugar (this will add about 8 grams carbohydrates per serving). Serve with toasted almonds for an extra shot of flavor and to reduce the overall glycemic index of the dessert.

Apricot-Orange Clafouti

172 calories, 25 g carbs

¼ cup granulated sugar
1 ⅓ cups 2% milk or unsweetened soy milk
¾ cup oat flour or whole grain pastry flour
¼ cup Splenda (a sugar substitute)
3 eggs
2 teaspoons grated orange peel
½ teaspoon grated ginger
½ teaspoon vanilla extract
2 cups (about 10) pitted and sliced apricots
¼ teaspoon ground cinnamon

Preheat the oven to 400°F. Coat a 9" deep-dish pie plate or quiche pan with cooking spray and dust with 1 teaspoon of the granulated sugar.

In a large bowl, whisk together the milk, flour, remaining sugar, Splenda, eggs, orange peel, ginger, and vanilla extract. Pour half of the batter into the prepared dish. Arrange the apricots evenly over the batter, then top with the remaining batter. Sprinkle with the cinnamon.

Bake for 40 minutes, or until puffed, browned, and firm. Cool on a rack for at least 15 minutes.

Makes 6 servings

Per serving: 172 calories, 8 g protein, 25 g carbohydrates, 5 g fat, 1 g saturated fat, 110 mg cholesterol, 3 g dietary fiber, 59 mg sodium

Diet exchanges: ½ milk, 0 vegetable, ½ fruit, ½ bread, ½ meat, ½ fat

Bread and Butter Pudding

323 calories, 35 g carbs

⅓ cup raisins
¼ cup whiskey or 1 teaspoon rum extract
2 cups 2% milk
⅓ cup heavy cream
¾ cup peach or apricot fruit spread
2 teaspoons vanilla extract
¾ teaspoon ground cinnamon
Pinch of salt
4 large eggs + 3 yolks, at room temperature
8 slices dried light whole wheat bread
3 tablespoons unsalted butter, softened
1 tablespoon confectioner's sugar (optional)

In a microwaveable cup or mug, combine the raisins and whiskey or rum extract. Microwave on high power until hot, 15 to 20 seconds. Cover to keep warm.

In a large saucepan, combine the milk, cream, fruit spread, vanilla extract, cinnamon, and salt. Cook over low heat until tiny bubbles appear around the edge of the pan, 8 to 10 minutes, stirring occasionally to incorporate the fruit spread.

Meanwhile, in a large bowl, whisk the eggs and yolks. Gradually whisk ½ cup of the milk mixture into the eggs. Quickly whisk in the remaining milk mixture. Strain the raisin-whiskey mixture over the egg mixture, reserving the raisins.

Coat an 8" × 8" baking pan with cooking spray. Spread 1 side of each bread slice with the butter. Cut the bread into cubes and arrange in the bottom of the prepared pan in an even layer. Scatter the raisins over the bread and pour the milk-egg mixture over the top.

Press a piece of plastic wrap directly onto the surface of the mixture. Let sit until the bread is thoroughly soaked, 30 to 40 minutes, occasionally pressing down on the plastic wrap to keep the bread submerged. Meanwhile, place a rack in the middle position in the oven and preheat the oven to 350°F.

Discard the plastic wrap and bake until a wooden skewer inserted in the center comes out clean, 45 to 50 minutes. Serve warm or at room temperature. Dust with the confectioner's sugar (if using).

Makes 8 servings

Per serving: 323 calories, 10 g protein, 35 g carbohydrates, 15 g fat, 7 g saturated fat, 215 mg cholesterol, 196 mg sodium, 1 g fiber

Diet exchanges: ½ milk, 0 vegetable, ½ fruit, 1½ bread, ½ meat, 2½ fat

PART V

Real People, Real Success

Losing Weight Meant No More Symptoms

Jennifer Byers, of Columbia, South Carolina, was diagnosed with diabetes in 1995. Despite her doctor's advice, she didn't take action until five years later, when she couldn't ignore her symptoms any longer. Heart palpitations, unquenchable thirst, and frequent nighttime trips to the bathroom finally convinced her that she needed to make some lifestyle changes.

Jennifer's first stop was the library, to learn more about her disease. That's when she began to understand how the combination of overweight, poor diet, and inactivity was definitely working against her. At the time, she weighed 225 pounds, was living on potato chips and pork chops, and wasn't getting any exercise. The case was clear-cut, and the verdict was in: Jennifer's unhealthy lifestyle had to go.

At first, she focused on getting more fiber and natural foods into her diet, since she had read that whole grains are absorbed more slowly and would help keep her blood sugar levels steady. She also replaced dinner entrées like red meat and ham with vegetable soup, and ate lots of bean burritos with onions and fresh peppers, muffins sweetened with bananas, and fresh fruit. She even found time, despite her hectic schedule with two kids, to bake her own whole wheat bread.

At last, Jennifer was following all the nutrition advice she had known for years. She was savoring squash, tomatoes, onions, and garlic from her garden instead of filling up on chips and baked goods from the grocery store.

Jennifer knew she had to exercise, too. The trouble was, she didn't like it. So she tried to make it as pleasant as possible. Instead of working out in the middle of a hot South Carolina day, she scheduled her sessions for 5:00 in the morning—when it was still cool, dark, and quiet outside. At first, she alternated between walking and running for a mile and a half. Soon she began looking for opportunities to be more active during the rest of the day. For example, rather than walking up stairs or to the mailbox, she'd run.

Jennifer's efforts paid off. In just three weeks, her symptoms disappeared. Within six months, she had lost 30 pounds and reclaimed the energy that diabetes had at first taken away.

Friendship Paved the Way to Successful Weight Loss

In 1994, Anita Beattie's doctor gave her a harsh ultimatum: "Lose weight, or don't come back to see me, because you're wasting my time and your money."

His words stung, but Anita knew that her doctor was right. She was too heavy for her height, and she had diabetes—a bad combination, to say the least. "He kicked me in my pants, and that's what I needed," says the Newport, Rhode Island, resident.

Determined to get in shape, Anita enrolled in a four-day hospital weight-loss program, where she learned the importance of eating better and exercising more. She began applying her new nutrition knowledge right away, making healthier food choices and controlling her portion sizes.

For exercise, Anita decided to try walking. But she knew that she'd need support—someone to prod her out the door when she felt like staying home. So she recruited some friends to join her. "Most of them are about my age, and like me, they want to stay active to keep themselves fit and healthy," she says.

Anita and her exercise buddies have established a

daily routine. They choose a time and place to meet, then set out for a brisk three-mile walk. For Anita, knowing that people are counting on her helps shake off any thoughts of skipping a workout. "Maybe it's a little cold or windy, or maybe I just don't feel like walking," she says. "I think of my friends waiting for me, and I don't want to leave them stranded."

When Anita goes to Florida for the winter, she doesn't leave her workout behind. She has exercise buddies there, too. Every day, they meet at 9:00 in the morning for a walk up and down the beach.

Anita's buddy-system approach to exercise helped her take off 38 pounds, which she has kept off for nine years. And with her doctor's guidance, she has successfully tapered off the insulin that she used to control her diabetes.

Mom Makes Her Health a Priority

Diabetes and heart disease had delivered a double whammy to Charlotte Libater. But she fought back with her own one-two punch: diet and exercise. Today, her will to win is keeping her active, involved, and cheerful against all odds.

Charlotte first found out she had type 2 diabetes some forty years ago. At the time, she was the struggling single mom of a 10-year-old boy, living in Charleston, South Carolina—the city she had adopted when first married. Her husband had died of a heart attack, leaving her as her son's sole provider.

And that worried her. Her son had already lost his dad. What would happen to him if she wasn't healthy?

Charlotte knew that she could help control her diabetes with a nutritious diet and exercise. So she indulged in heaping helpings of steamed vegetables and turned to fish, chicken, and turkey for her protein. With her office not even a mile away from home, she walked to work every day. "The best part was that I felt so much better," she says.

Even with the most vigilant care, however, diabetes

can be an insidious disease. Within twenty years, Charlotte became insulin-dependent. She learned to give herself insulin shots every day. Then another health setback: On February 10, 1991—she remembers it as if it were yesterday—she suffered a heart attack.

As scared as Charlotte was, she mustered the courage to bounce back, thanks to some reassuring words from her surgeon. Charlotte had survived, the surgeon said, because she had taken such good care of herself. Her immune system was strong. And she needed to keep it that way.

Charlotte joined a hospital cardiac rehabilitation program. To this day, she goes three times a week to work out on the treadmill and the stationary and recumbent bicycles. "I still watch my diet, and I check my blood sugar levels twice a day," she says.

While she attributes her renewed health to her lifestyle, Charlotte contends that she would not feel as good about herself were she not involved in so many activities in the community and her synagogue. She volunteers with the Charleston chapter of Mended Hearts, a nonprofit support group for heart disease patients and their families; she sings in choirs, including the Jewish Choral Society; and she is a volunteer usher for the Charleston Symphony and the Dock Street Theatre.

"I force myself to rest every afternoon, to sit quietly and read. I haven't much energy or time left for housework, so I do as little as I can," she says happily. "I realize that I can take care of my health, no matter what the obstacles."

She Traded Her Candy Bars for a Treadmill

Sylvia Charity knows diabetes all too well. Both type 1 and type 2 run in her family. Her mother died from complications of the disease.

So when Sylvia first noticed diabetes' telltale signs—frequent bathroom trips, raging thirst, light-headedness—she immediately asked her doctor to check her blood sugar. Her worst fear was confirmed: She had type 2 diabetes. "At first, I was heartbroken," she says. "But then I became very angry because I felt responsible for allowing my fear to become a reality."

Like many women her age, Sylvia—a government supervisor from Hampton, Virginia—had put on some weight over the years. She had slacked off on exercise, spending most of her days confined to a desk at work. "After always being able to do whatever I wanted, like eating a piece of cake or a banana split, I finally realized I was going to have to adjust my life," she says. "It felt like the end of the world at the time, but now I know I can live with it."

Sylvia, who describes herself as a chocoholic,

stopped buying candy bars. She cut back on high-carbohydrate meals, and she made a point of balancing the carbs she did eat with small portions of meat and vegetables. With her doctor's approval, she started working out on a treadmill three or four times a week. She's up to twenty-five minutes a session.

So far, Sylvia has lost 23 pounds, and she keeps her blood sugar pretty much in check. "This is not an overnight thing," she notes. "Temptation is all around. But I've got six grandkids that I want to see grow up. I know I need to keep my priorities straight and stay in control of my life."

Taking the First Step toward Blood Sugar Control

Environmental health specialist Jacqueline Bellinger was just a few months shy of her thirty-ninth birthday when she was diagnosed with type 2 diabetes. Blood tests showed a fasting blood sugar of 263, more than double the 126 that's considered diabetic.

For Jacqueline, the news didn't come as a big surprise. After all, diabetes—both type 1 and type 2—seems to run in her family. And she knew that she weighed more than she should, carrying 310 pounds on her 5-foot-9 frame.

She wasted no time embarking on a diet-and-exercise regimen that ultimately took off 152 pounds and changed her life for the better. "I met with a diabetes educator and nutritionist," she explains. "The first thing we did was empty the larder at home. A few of my friends and relatives made out handsomely with Polish sausage and 12-ounce steaks. After about six months, I lost my taste for foods like rich meats. I would rather just eat a little lean meat and fill up on vegetables."

Once Jacqueline launched a walking program—

thirty minutes a day, every day—the pounds quickly melted away. But because walking isn't always practical in her neck of the woods (eastern Washington), especially during the winter, she added cross-country ski machines and stationary bikes to her fitness routine. "I use an exercise machine for forty-five minutes in the morning and thirty minutes before going to bed at night," she says. "And I like to walk a lot when I'm on vacation. In fact, a vacation isn't any fun without it!"

These days, Jacqueline's blood sugar hovers in the near-normal range. She continues to work hard to eat healthful foods and exercise regularly, because she wants to protect her body from the complications that diabetes can cause. "I've seen these complications firsthand, in members of my father's family. Two of my uncles ended up blind," she explains. "I'm not getting off scot-free, either. I already have some kidney damage. But if I keep my blood sugar at a near-normal level, I can reduce my chances of developing further complications. So far, I don't need pills."

Her efforts continue to pay off. "I feel so much better now. When you feel better physically, you feel better emotionally," Jacqueline says. "It's great fun going shopping, too. They didn't make large-size clothes for teenagers in the 1970s. Now I'm wearing all the fun stuff I didn't wear years ago: tie-dyes and flared jeans."

PART VI

Resources

To Learn More

If you've ever tried searching for trustworthy diabetes information on the Internet, you may have felt a bit overwhelmed by all that's out there. Next time, you might want start by checking out one of these reliable sources. (As you'll see, we've also included phone numbers, in case you prefer to call an organization instead.)

American Diabetes Association (ADA)
Web site: www.diabetes.org
Tel: (703) 549-1500 or (800) DIABETES (342-2383); to order publications, (800) 232-6733
Among the Web site's special features are search tools to help locate qualified physicians and diabetes education programs in your area.

Centers for Disease Control and Prevention (CDC)
Web site: www.cdc.gov/diabetes
E-mail: diabetes@cdc.gov
Tel: (877) CDC-DIAB (232-3422)
The Web site offers fact sheets, statistics, publications, and information about state diabetes control programs.

Joslin Diabetes Center
Web site: www.joslin.org
Tel: (617) 732-2400 or (800) JOSLIN-1 (567-5461)
The center publishes the quarterly newsletter *Joslin*, as well as books, videotapes, and other educational materials for diabetes patients and health-care professionals.

Juvenile Diabetes Research Foundation International (JDF)
Web site: www.jdf.org
E-mail: info@jdf.org
Tel: (800) JDF-CURE (533-2873) or (212) 785-9500
Among the JDF's publications are the quarterly journal *Countdown*, the quarterly newsletter *Research News*, and a series of patient-education brochures for those with type 1 or type 2 diabetes.

National Diabetes Information Clearinghouse (NDIC)
Web site: www.niddk.nih.gov/health/diabetes/ndic.htm
E-mail: ndic@info.niddk.nih.gov
Tel: (800) 860-8747 or (301) 654-3327
The NDIC offers diabetes education materials for free or for a nominal fee, as well as a quarterly newsletter for health-care professionals.

Index